welcome
pages 6-7

how to use
pages 8-9

at a glance
pages 10-13

meet the specialists
pages 14-17

allergens in children
pages 18-33

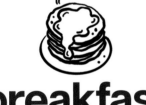

breakfast
pages 35-63

lunch +
snacks
pages 65-105

dinner
pages 107-151

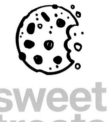

sweet
treats
pages 153-189

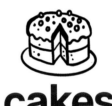

cakes
pages 191-215

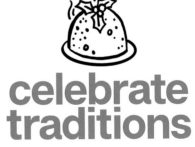

celebrate
traditions
pages 217-243

index
pages 244-252

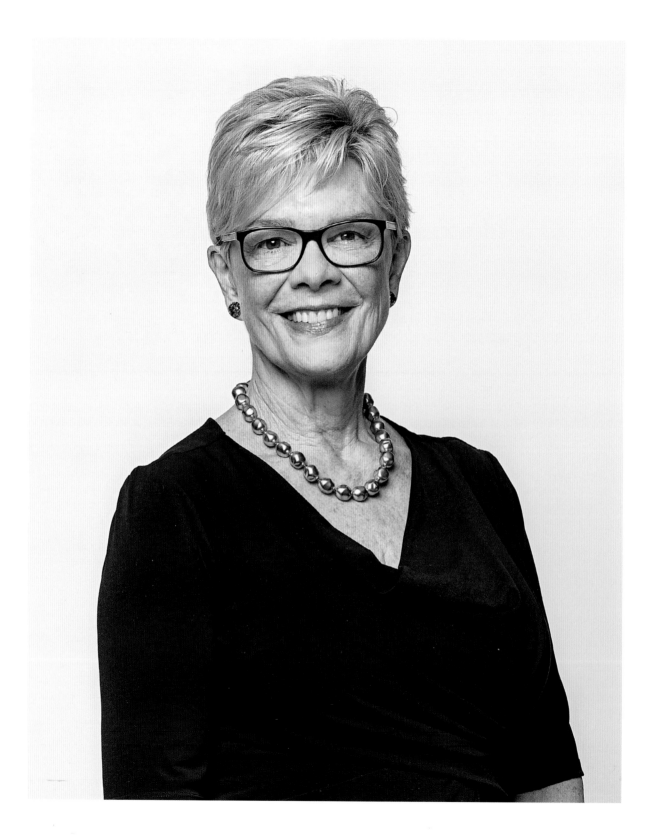

The Allergy Friendly
Family Cookbook

Expert advice from world-leading child allergy specialists
at Murdoch Children's Research Institute
and 100+ recipes from Australia's No.1 food site

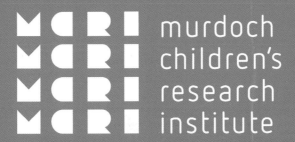

MCRI murdoch
MCRI children's
MCRI research
MCRI institute

contents

welcome

Australia is unenviably known as the 'allergy capital of the world'. With more than five million of us living with allergies, it is clear many families will find this book an invaluable addition to their cookbook collection.

At Murdoch Children's Research Institute, our work aims to ensure that children live in a world defined by wellness rather than by illness. We want every child to live a healthy and fulfilled life. Furthermore, we want families and their communities to prosper.

It is this purpose, combined with our relentless determination to tackle the toughest issues affecting child health, which makes me immensely proud to lead the Institute. As Australia's largest child health research institute – comprising more than 1400 curious and clever researchers and clinicians – we are very excited to see this collection of recipes come to life for children and their caregivers. To ensure our efforts are long-lasting and wide-reaching, our focus is on prevention and early intervention, rather than waiting for disease to occur and then trying to treat it. We are pushing traditional boundaries by investing in digital technologies informed by rigorous medical science to make healthcare more accessible, and we strive to ensure equitable outcomes for disadvantaged children both locally and abroad.

Murdoch Children's has also recently embarked on one of the world's largest and most ambitious longitudinal studies of a generation, called 'GenV'. GenV will study up to 100,000 children born in Victoria, Australia, along with their parents, following their health for the rest of their lives. Not only will we be able to track the frequency of illnesses, such as allergy and asthma, but we will be able to introduce new prevention strategies and interventions in real time.

I am very proud of all those involved, and appreciative of our many partners and generous donors who support us on our journey of discovery. And I am just as thankful to the many children, families and communities who participate in our research activities, working with us to achieve remarkable outcomes that will be felt today and for many generations to come.

To deliver projects that have wide-scale impact on child health, our community participants are our greatest allies. Whether they are involved in a clinical trial of a new treatment, contributing samples to a research project or helping to develop clinical and community guidelines, our work is made possible through the strong partnerships we hold – especially with families like yours.

Best wishes,

Professor Kathryn North AC
DIRECTOR,
MURDOCH CHILDREN'S
RESEARCH INSTITUTE

how to use

The Allergy Friendly
Family Cookbook

Welcome to 100+ family-friendly recipes, tips and at-a-glance icons – everything you need to cook meals, sweets and snacks allergy friendly and carefree!

amazing features

Colour-coded chapters

ALLERGY-FREE ICONS
Our coloured icons indicate Egg Free, Dairy Free, Nut Free, Sesame Free, Gluten and Wheat Free, Soy Free, Fish and Shellfish Free meals

Helpful prep and cooking times

Complete nutritional information

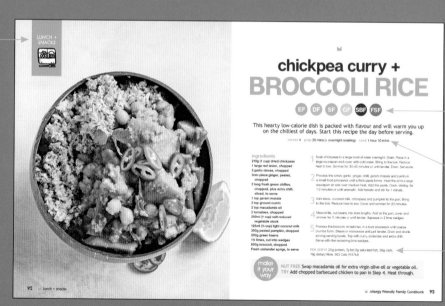

chickpea curry + BROCCOLI RICE

EF DF SF GF SBF FSF

This hearty low-calorie dish is packed with flavour and will warm you up on the chilliest of days. Start this recipe the day before serving.

serves 4   prep 20 mins (+ overnight soaking)   cook 1 hour 10 mins

ingredients
210g (1 cup) dried chickpeas
1 large red onion, chopped
3 garlic cloves, chopped
3cm-piece ginger, peeled, chopped
2 long fresh green chillies, chopped, plus extra chilli, sliced, to serve
1 tsp garam masala
2 tsp ground cumin
2 tsp macadamia oil
2 tomatoes, chopped
250ml (1 cup) salt-reduced vegetable stock
125ml (½ cup) light coconut milk
300g peeled pumpkin, chopped
200g green beans
1½ limes, cut into wedges
600g broccoli, chopped
Fresh coriander sprigs, to serve

1. Soak chickpeas in a large bowl of water overnight. Drain. Place in a large saucepan and cover with cold water. Bring to the boil. Reduce heat to low. Simmer for 30-40 minutes or until tender. Drain. Set aside.

2. Process the onion, garlic, ginger, chilli, garam masala and cumin in a small food processor until a thick paste forms. Heat the oil in a large saucepan or wok over medium heat. Add the paste. Cook, stirring, for 1-2 minutes or until aromatic. Add tomato and stir for 1 minute.

3. Add stock, coconut milk, chickpeas and pumpkin to the pan. Bring to the boil. Reduce heat to low. Cover and simmer for 20 minutes.

4. Meanwhile, cut beans into 4cm lengths. Add to the pan, cover and simmer for 5 minutes or until tender. Squeeze in 2 lime wedges.

5. Process the broccoli, in batches, in a food processor until coarse crumbs form. Steam or microwave until just tender. Drain and divide among serving bowls. Top with curry, coriander and extra chilli. Serve with the remaining lime wedges.

PER SERVE 25g protein, 7g fat (3g saturated fat), 34g carb, 19g dietary fibre, 363 Cals (1517kJ)

make it your way
NUT FREE Swap macadamia oil for extra virgin olive oil or vegetable oil.
TRY Add chopped barbecued chicken to pan in Step 4. Heat through.

92 lunch + snacks

Allergy Friendly Family Cookbook 93

allergy-free icons

We want your daily meal and snack prep to be as stress-free as possible. With easy colour-coded icons, you can immediately see which recipes fulfil your dietary needs. Take a look at our 'Make It Your Way' section under each recipe for ways to adapt recipes to cater for even more allergies.

 Egg Free

 Sesame Free

 Soy Free

 Dairy Free

 Gluten + Wheat Free

 Fish + Shellfish Free

 Nut Free

INDEX

Our index is designed in three ways, so you can easily find the dishes you'd like to cook for yourself and the family. Search by alphabetical order, browse via the seven main allergens, plus their 'Make it Your Way' options, and look up a dish by a key ingredient. Deciding what to cook has never been easier!

Allergy Friendly Family Cookbook
ALPHABETICAL INDEX

Allergy Friendly Family Cookbook
INDEX BY ALLERGEN

MAKE IT YOUR WAY Change the recipe to suit your allergy-free needs. Plus, helpful recipe boosts and tips.

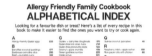

DAIRY FREE Swap the natural yoghurt for dairy-free coconut yoghurt.
NUT FREE Omit the almonds and serve with chopped fruit, if desired.

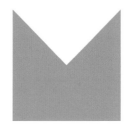

at a glance

Choosing your daily meals and snacks is easy with 'at a glance', which provides a snapshot of all the recipes in this cookbook. Use our colour-coded icons to instantly see which ones fulfil your dietary needs. Many recipes have extra allergy-friendly options – you'll find these in our index, from page 244.

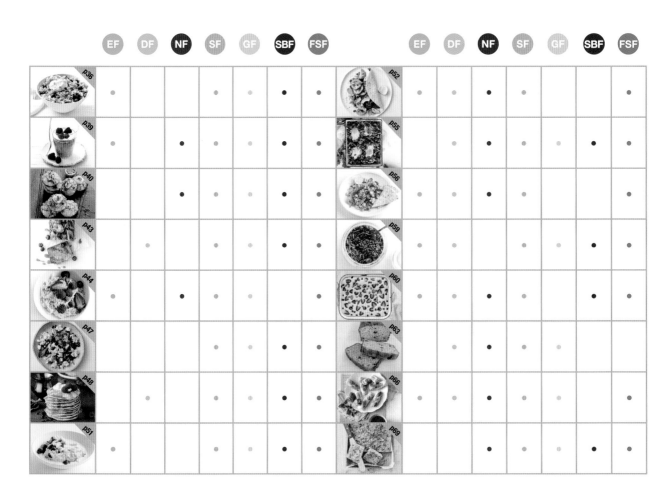

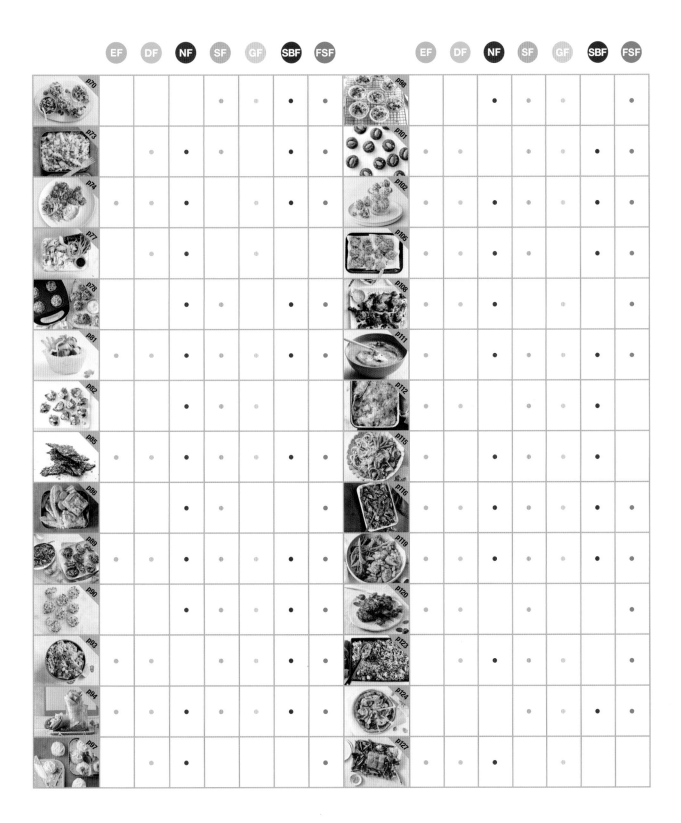

Page	EF	DF	NF	SF	GF	SBF	FSF
p70				○	○	●	●
p73		○	●	●		●	●
p74	○	○	●	○	○	●	●
p77		○	●		○		
p78			●			●	●
p81	○	○	●	○	○	●	●
p82			●	○			
p85	○	○	●	○	○	●	●
p86			●	○			●
p89	○	○	●	○		●	●
p90			●	○	○	●	●
p93	○	○		○	○	●	●
p94	○	○	●	○		●	●
p97		○	●				●

Page	EF	DF	NF	SF	GF	SBF	FSF
p98			●	○	○		○
p101	○	○		○	○	●	●
p102	○	○	●	○	○	●	●
p105	○	○	●	○	○	●	●
p108	○		●		○		○
p111	○		●	●	○	●	●
p112	●	○	●	○	○	●	
p115	○		●	○	○	●	●
p116	○	○	●	○	○	●	●
p119	○	○	●	○	○	●	●
p120	○	○		○	○		●
p123		○	●	○	○		●
p124					○	●	
p127	○	○	●		○		

	EF	DF	NF	SF	GF	SBF	FSF		EF	DF	NF	SF	GF	SBF	FSF
p128	•	•	•	•	•	•	•	p158	•			•	•	•	•
p131	•	•		•		•	•	p161	•		•	•	•	•	•
p132	•		•	•		•	•	p162	•			•	•	•	•
p135	•	•	•	•	•			p165		•		•	•		•
p136	•	•	•	•			•	p166	•	•	•	•	•	•	•
p139	•	•	•	•	•	•	•	p169	•	•	•	•	•	•	•
p140	•	•	•	•	•	•	•	p170	•	•	•	•	•	•	•
p143	•	•		•			•	p173	•	•	•	•			•
p144	•		•	•	•	•	•	p174	•	•	•	•	•	•	•
p147	•		•	•	•	•	•	p177	•	•	•	•	•	•	•
p148	•	•	•	•	•	•	•	p178	•	•	•	•	•	•	•
p151	•	•	•	•			•	p181	•	•	•	•	•	•	•
p154			•	•	•	•	•	p182	•	•	•	•	•	•	•
p157	•	•			•	•	•	p185	•	•	•	•		•	•

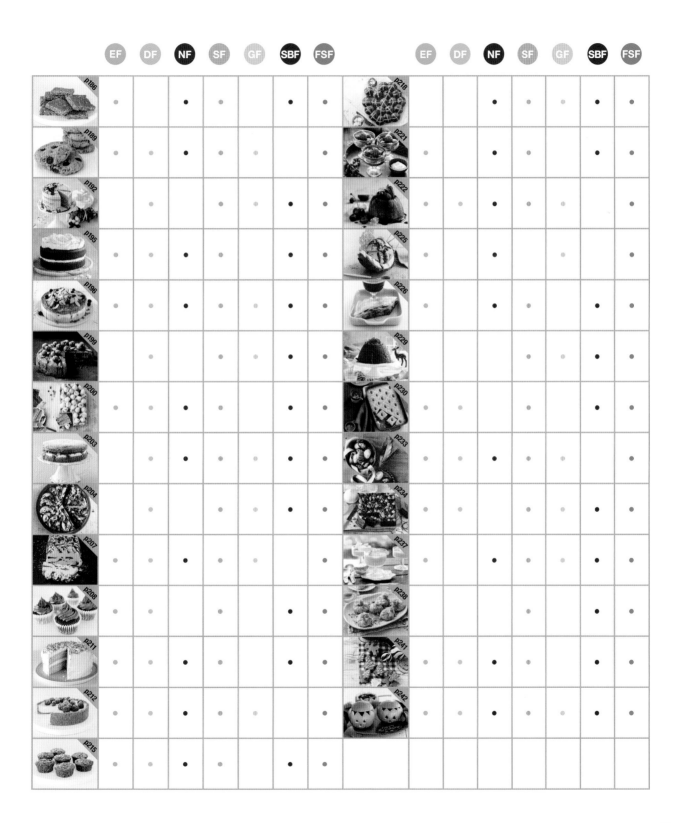

	EF	DF	NF	SF	GF	SBF	FSF		EF	DF	NF	SF	GF	SBF	FSF
p186	○		●	○		●	●	p218			●	○	○	●	●
p189	○	○	●	○	○		●	p221	○		●	○		●	●
p192		○	○	○	○	●	●	p222	○		●	○	○		●
p195	○	○	●	○		●	●	p225	○		●		○		●
p196	○	○	●	○	○	●	●	p226	○		●	○		●	●
p199		○	○	○	○	●	●	p229				○	○	●	●
p200	○	○	●	○		●	●	p230	○	○		○		●	●
p203		○	●	○	○	●	○	p233	○	○	●	○	○		●
p204		○	○	○	○	●	●	p234	○	○		○	○	●	●
p207	○	○	●	○	○		●	p237	○		●	○	○	●	●
p208	○	○	○	○		●	●	p238						●	●
p211	○	○	●	○		●	●	p241	○	○	●	○		●	●
p212	○	○	●	○	○		●	p242	○	○	●	○	○	●	●
p215	○	○	●	○		●	●								

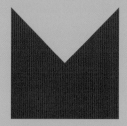

meet the specialists

Allergy research is constantly evolving. At the forefront of this research is the Murdoch Children's Research Institute. Get to know Mimi, Kirsten and Vicki, who are tirelessly striving to optimise the wellbeing of families living with allergies.

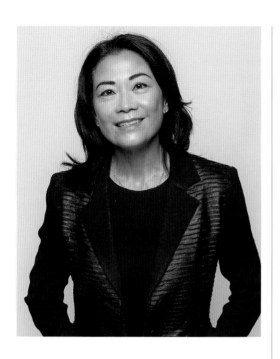

For families living with food allergies,

cooking meals at home offers a way to keep children safe. However, recipes are often difficult to navigate and allergen-free recipes specific to a family's needs are hard to find. Trying to decipher (or find!) ingredient lists to see if allergens are present can be time-consuming, confusing and understandably anxiety-inducing.

As a paediatric allergist immunologist at Murdoch Children's Research Institute, I am pleased to contribute to this book, which shows how you and your family can eat well, and safely, while eliminating relevant food allergens from your daily meals. It brings together the discoveries we have made to support those living with allergies.

As a researcher – and clinician – my work centres around freeing children and families from the burden of living with food allergy. My goal is to offer immediate solutions that reduce fear, anxiety and distress for allergic children and their families, and develop future treatments that will let children live allergy free.

My work centres around freeing children and families from the burden of living with food allergy.

My research team at Murdoch Children's has spent two decades developing novel immunotherapy treatments that induce remission of peanut allergy. A 200-patient trial showed these treatments led to the highest remission rates ever reported in school-aged children, allowing them to enjoy substantial improvement in their quality of life.

We are also developing innovative tools to keep allergic children safe in the care of others. This work also aims to reduce stress and fear surrounding allergic reactions, which better empowers children living with allergy along with their community of carers. These tools lead to more impactful self-management, and I'm excited this book will add to this work.

This book provides an easy guide to preparing snacks and meals for loved ones living with food allergies. We've included tips on adapting meals to cater to your child from infancy and childhood, through to the independence of young adulthood.

I hope this book will make mealtimes a positive experience for all to enjoy!

Mimi

Professor Mimi Tang
MBBS, PHD, FRACP, FRCPA, FAAAAI
Head of Allergy Immunology Research Group and Director of Allergy Translation at Murdoch Children's Research Institute
Professorial Fellow, Department of Paediatrics, University of Melbourne
Consultant Allergist and Immunologist, The Royal Children's Hospital

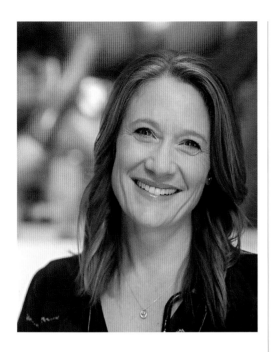

When my children were young,

I would have loved an allergy-friendly cookbook. Two of my daughters had a cow's milk allergy and I will never forget living with the anxiety that, at any time, potentially with the next snack or meal, my child might have a severe reaction.

On average, one child in every classroom will have a food allergy. My vision is that one day no child will have to go to school with a food allergy. It is an ambitious goal, but we are making significant inroads.

At Murdoch Children's Research Institute, we have conducted large studies with more than 16,000 children – HealthNuts, EarlyNuts and SchoolNuts – to enhance our understanding of the risk factors and consequences of food allergy. The results are helping inform changes to food allergy prevention, diagnosis and management.

The HealthNuts team study found up to 10 per cent of Australian infants have a confirmed food allergy. Hospital data also indicates a rapid increase in food allergy.

My vision is that one day no child will have to go to school with a food allergy.

Our team also showed that introducing egg early in life can help prevent egg allergy. This research, combined with results from peanut studies, led to the development of consensus infant feeding guidelines recommending allergenic solid foods in the first year of life, which is now adopted across Australia and the world. Since then, we have started to see a decrease in peanut allergy among infants.

There are five main risk factors for food allergies, which our research defined. Coined 'the 5Ds', these include diet, dry skin, vitamin D, dogs (external environmental exposure) and dribble (gut microbiome).

Together with researchers and clinicians around Australia, we are conducting large trials to assess whether additional strategies can prevent food allergies in infants. These approaches include different levels of allergenic foods in the diet during pregnancy, skin barrier creams or vaccines in early life, along with infant vitamin supplementation.

Our team is also leading some exciting trials assessing strategies to treat food allergies in young children, at a time when the immune system seems to be more responsive to change.

I look forward to sharing our results with you. In the meantime, enjoy preparing these allergy-friendly recipes. I know I will.

Kirsten

Associate Professor Kirsten Perrett
MBBS, FRACP, PHD
Head of Population Allergy Research Group and Deputy Director of the Melbourne Children's Trial Centre at Murdoch Children's Research Institute
Principal Fellow, Department of Paediatrics, The University of Melbourne
Consultant Allergist and Vaccinologist, The Royal Children's Hospital

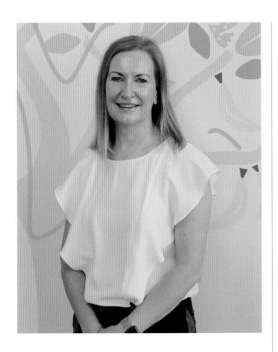

Juggling food allergies, especially multiple food allergies, can be challenging, and that's why I am so excited to be a part of this book. The information and recipes within go a long way to alleviating that daily anxiety many people feel when dealing with allergy and trying to prepare meals. These recipes are safe and they are tasty enough that the whole family can enjoy them together – one of the most frequent requests we receive.

When I first meet families in the allergy clinic embarking on their food allergy journey, it can be a scary and overwhelming time for them. This is a medical condition that affects whole families, not just those with the allergy.

As a specialist allergy dietician, I am part of the research team at Murdoch Children's Research Institute exploring dietary interventions to prevent and treat food allergies. It gives me immense satisfaction being able to help families identify their child's allergen in foods, recipes and commercial food products – as well as helping them to ensure they know how to get replacement foods to keep their child's diet nutritionally adequate. My passion is to arm the family with shopping and cooking skills that will allow children with allergies to have the same positive experiences around food that many of us take for granted. It is my hope that all children with allergies can enjoy the same things in life as those without allergies – eating together as a family, going to parties, having a birthday cake, heading off to a school camp or sleepover.

I am sure the recipes in this cookbook will become new family favourites and, together with Mimi and Kirsten and the research team at Murdoch Children's Research Institute, we look forward to sharing the results of all our ongoing research with you soon.

It is my hope that all children with allergies can enjoy the same things in life as those without allergies.

Vicki

Dr Vicki McWilliam
B.SCI. MND PHD ADV APD
Research Officer, Population Allergy Research Group
Murdoch Children's Research Institute
Senior Allergy Dietitian, Department of Allergy and Immunology, The Royal Children's Hospital
Honorary Senior Research Fellow, Department of Paediatrics, Faculty of Medicine Dentistry and Health Sciences, University of Melbourne

most common allergens in children

Some allergies are outgrown and some are there to stay. Here is a little insight into the top seven.

In this book, you'll find recipes that are safe and delicious for children allergic to the seven most common allergens in Australia. Those allergens are:

1. egg
2. dairy (cow's and other animals' milks)
3. nuts (peanut and tree nuts)
4. sesame
5. gluten and wheat
6. soy
7. fish and shellfish.

Egg

Almost 10 per cent of babies have an allergy to egg. Most children grow out of this allergy by the time they are four years old, and many more will outgrow their egg allergy by the time they are a teen.

If your child cannot tolerate cooked egg, they may still be able to eat egg that is baked in a product, such as egg baked in muffins, cakes or biscuits. It's best to speak with your doctor or allergist about whether it's safe and appropriate to try these foods with your child.

Almost 10% of babies have an allergy to egg. Most children grow out of this allergy.

Dairy

An allergy to cow's milk affects around 1.5 per cent of babies at 12 months of age. Most children will grow out of this allergy but studies suggest it may take longer to outgrow it, and many children can remain allergic to milk into their teen years.

Being allergic to cow's milk usually means also avoiding other dairy products and milk from other animals such as sheep and goats. It's important to have clear direction from your doctor about what foods your child should be avoiding.

Children without a milk allergy may still suffer lactose intolerance, which is when the body doesn't produce enough lactase, an enzyme that helps digest lactose, the sugar in milk. It's not dangerous – it doesn't cause a rash or anaphylaxis – but it can lead to diarrhoea, vomiting, stomach pain and gas.

If your child cannot tolerate milk or dairy products, they may be able to eat small amounts baked into muffins, cakes or biscuits. Speak to your doctor or allergist about whether this is safe for your child.

Nuts and seeds

Peanut allergy is the most common nut allergy in children and babies, with almost 3 per cent having a peanut allergy at the age of 12 months. Allergies can also occur to 'tree nuts' such as almonds, brazil nuts, cashews, hazelnuts, macadamia nuts, pecans, pine nuts, pistachios and walnuts; and also to seeds such as sesame.

While peanut, tree nuts and seeds are different plant families, it is not uncommon for people to be allergic to more than one nut or seed. Around one-third of those with an allergy to peanut will go on to have allergies to other nuts. Work with your doctor to find out which nuts are safe to include in your child's diet, and how you can introduce them.

Most children who are allergic to nuts or seeds will have that allergy for life, although some (around 30 per cent, in the case of peanut) may grow out of it by early school years. Although it may be easier to eliminate nuts or sesame seed from your child's diet over other allergens, allergic reactions due to accidental exposure can still happen and reactions can be severe. Peanut and tree nuts are two of the most common causes of life-threatening anaphylaxis, and reactions can be due to small traces of the proteins.

Gluten and wheat

A wheat allergy is an immune response to one or more of the proteins in wheat. This is different to coeliac disease where there's an intolerance to gluten. Gluten is one of the proteins in wheat, which is why you often see wheat and gluten allergies spoken about interchangeably. But someone allergic to wheat could be allergic to another protein in wheat other than gluten. And gluten is found in grains other than wheat, such as barley, rye and standard oats (note, gluten-free oats are available), so it's important to know the difference if you're trying to avoid a particular allergen.

Around one-third of those with an allergy to peanut will go on to have allergies to other nuts.

Some children who have a wheat allergy when they're young may grow out of it, and some may develop the allergy later in life.

Soybean

While a soy allergy isn't as common as some other childhood allergies, soy is present in many packaged foods, so it can be difficult to avoid. It's important to always check the ingredient label on foods, and to ask at restaurants before ordering, to ensure your child isn't consuming hidden soy.

Most children with a soy allergy will outgrow it by the time they are an adult.

Fish and shellfish

An allergy to fish or shellfish may not seem too difficult to manage in children – lobster isn't usually on the menu for most families! But it's important to avoid cross-contamination when foods are prepared in the same space as shellfish.

Shellfish can be divided into two families: molluscs (abalone, clams, cockles, limpets, pipis, mussels, squid/calamari, octopus, scallops and snails), and crustaceans (crabs, lobsters, prawns, crayfish, bugs, and yabbies). Some children will be allergic to just one family and others allergic to all shellfish.

Around 1 per cent of the population has a shellfish allergy, and it is usually lifelong. Many children who have this allergy can still eat canned fish without a reaction, as long as it is not prepared near any shellfish.

Note: For a list of foods containing your child's allergen, plus alternatives, visit the Australian Society of Clinical Immunology and Allergy (ASCIA) via this QR code.

about allergens in children

Get to know more about allergy triggers, allergic reactions, and how you can manage food in your child's life.

Any substance that is harmless for most people, but that triggers an allergic immune reaction in some, is called an allergen. In a person who is allergic, their immune system mistakenly sees that allergen as a threat, and causes an allergic reaction when they are exposed to that allergen.

Common allergens that can trigger an allergic reaction are:

- inhaled allergens such as dust mites, pet dander, pollen or mould spores
- foods such as egg, milk or nuts
- insect stings from bees, wasps, or certain types of ants
- medicines.

About one in ten babies, as well as 4-8 per cent of children under the age of five, have some type of food allergy. Usually, an allergic response happens very quickly, but it can take up to an hour. Most reactions are mild, but when they involve the breathing or circulation, they can be life threatening.

Food allergy can be scary for parents, and challenging to manage, especially when trying to get used to reading food labels and handling social occasions. However, managing your child's allergy does get easier over time. Our goal

Many children will grow out of their allergies naturally.

with this book is to provide accurate evidence-based information that's easy to refer to at any time.

There is no cure for food allergy, but many children will grow out of their allergies naturally. In the meantime, the only way to avoid a reaction is to help your child to avoid the allergen.

About allergic reactions

There are two types of food allergy: one causes reactions shortly after eating the food (known as an IgE-mediated food allergy), and the other can cause delayed reactions hours after eating the food (known as a non-IgE-mediated food allergy).

IgE-mediated food allergy

Most people are familiar with the immediate type of food allergy. These allergies usually cause reactions within minutes of eating the food.

Common symptoms are:

- hives
- swelling of the lips, eyes or face
- difficulty breathing.

This type of allergy causes anaphylaxis – a life-threatening reaction affecting a person's breathing and/or circulation.

Non-IgE-mediated food allergy

Delayed food allergies are less well known. They usually cause gut symptoms, such as vomiting, tummy pain and/or diarrhoea, several hours or days after eating the food. This type of food allergy doesn't cause anaphylaxis, although it can sometimes lead to circulation problems. The lag in symptoms presenting themselves can make it more difficult to figure out what has caused your child's allergic symptoms.

If you think your child may be allergic to something, whether their reaction is mild or more severe, immediate or delayed, it's important for them to be properly assessed so you know what they are allergic to, and you can learn how to manage their allergy.

Your family doctor can help to assess your child and organise a blood test, or they may refer you to a paediatrician or allergy specialist for further testing.

Skin-prick test

Immunoglobuin (IgE) antibodies are proteins that the immune system usually makes to eliminate parasites. In people without allergies, IgE antibodies are usually only present at low levels. However, in people with IgE-mediated allergies, the immune system makes IgE antibodies against the allergen, which then cause an allergic reaction to the allergen.

To diagnose an IgE-mediated allergy, your doctor can test for the presence of IgE antibodies against the allergen by performing a skin-prick test or a blood test.

A skin-prick test is where the skin is pricked with a device that looks a little bit like a toothpick, and contains a drop of a suspected allergen. If your child's skin reacts by swelling and/or turning red, the test is considered positive. Skin-prick tests are quick and easy, and despite their scary name, aren't very painful.

Skin-prick tests are only useful for diagnosing the immediate type of food allergy (IgE) and are used to confirm an

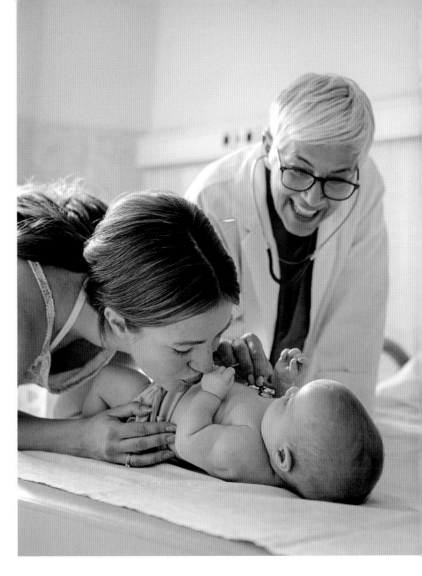

> If you think your child may be allergic to something, it is important for them to be properly assessed.

allergy that is already suspected because there was a reaction to the food. They are not used to screen for a possible allergy when your child hasn't eaten the food yet, because they can often be positive even when a child is not allergic to the food.

Blood test

A blood test can also detect IgE-mediated food allergies.

Like skin-prick tests, blood tests are only useful for diagnosing the immediate type of food allergy, and are used to confirm an allergy that is already suspected. Allergy blood tests are not used to screen for a possible allergy when a child hasn't eaten the food yet, as they are often positive even when the child is not allergic to the food.

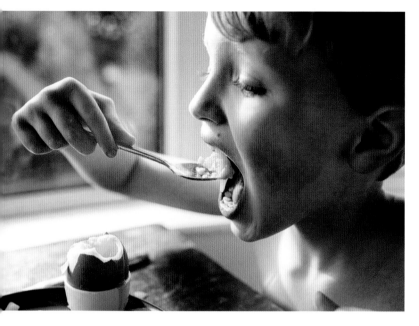

Oral food challenge

Your doctor may recommend an oral food challenge to confirm a diagnosis of food allergy. This involves your child being given small and increasing amounts of a suspected allergen in a supervised clinical setting. They are observed while eating the food and then for some time afterwards to see how their body responds to the food.

A word about alternative therapies and testing: There are many allergy tests and treatments offered by unorthodox or alternative therapists that are not regulated by government or based on medical evidence. The Australasian Society of Clinical Immunology and Allergy (ASCIA) recommends consulting a qualified medical practitioner for any suspected food allergy.

Mild allergic reaction

Allergic reactions can vary in severity. Your child may suffer from a mild allergic reaction. The symptoms may include:
- a rash, welts or hives
- swelling of the face, eyes or lips

As your child starts to grow up, feed themselves and make food choices without you, it's important to teach them to manage their food allergy.

- an itchy or tingling mouth
- diarrhoea, stomach pain or vomiting.

Anaphylaxis

A child may have a more severe reaction to an allergen, known as anaphylaxis, can be life threatening.

Symptoms of anaphylaxis may include:
- difficulty breathing
- noisy breathing
- swelling of the tongue and/or throat
- hoarse voice or difficulty talking
- wheezing or a persistent cough
- dizziness or fainting
- a young child going pale or floppy.

An anaphylactic reaction will usually happen 20-60 minutes after your child has eaten their allergen. It's important to always treat anaphylaxis as a medical emergency.

Immediate treatment with adrenaline, delivered by an injector, such as an EpiPen or Anapen, is usually recommended. EpiPens and Anapens are easy to use and, if your child has had one prescribed, it should be carried at all times.

If your child has any of these symptoms, stop giving them the food immediately and talk to your doctor about treatment.

Teaching children how to manage their own allergies

As your child starts to grow up and make food choices without your supervision, it's important to teach them, in an age-appropriate way, to manage their own food allergy. This is the best way to keep them safe, because they won't always be under your careful watch. Ensure they know:

1. what foods they are allergic to, how it affects them, and what to do about it if they have a reaction.
2. how to explain politely and clearly what they can and can't eat, and why it's important.
3. to ask what is in foods before they eat them, and to understand ways their allergen might be present in foods that may not be obvious.

4. how to read food labels and understand that the way a food is prepared might affect whether they can eat it.
5. that the safest approach is to not eat a food if they are unsure it is safe for them to eat.
6. not to share someone else's food at school or anywhere else.

Maintaining a balanced diet while avoiding specific allergens

Many of the common food allergens are from core food groups in our diet, and the removal of these allergens can have an impact on nutrition if we don't include suitable substitutes.

Many common food allergens are from core food groups in our diet, which can impact nutrition.

If you're eliminating a particular food from your child's diet, it can mean it's eliminated from the entire family. However, it only takes a few tweaks to be sure your everyday diet keeps everyone healthy. It's true, some allergens may be present in lots of foods, making them difficult to avoid, but it's important to ensure your child eats enough foods from these five recognised food groups every day.

1. vegetables
2. fruit
3. grain foods (mostly whole grains)
4. dairy and dairy alternatives
5. proteins: lean meat and poultry, fish, eggs, tofu, nuts, seeds and legumes

The table below outlines the essential nutrients that are found in common allergens, and suitable alternatives.

Food allergen	Nutrients in this food	Suitable alternatives
Egg	Protein and iron	Meat, fish and nuts
Dairy	Protein, carbohydrate, fat, calcium, vitamin D, vitamin B12 and iodine	Plant-based milk substitutes, yoghurts and cheese (look for products with added calcium). For infants under 12 months, specialised infant formula should be used.
Nuts and seeds	Protein, carbohydrate, fat, fibre and iron	Meat, fish and eggs
Wheat and gluten	Carbohydrate, fibre and folate	Other grain sources, but be aware that some are forms of wheat or hybrids of wheat.
Soy	Protein, fat and fibre	Isolated soy allergy has minimal impact, if excluded.
Fish and shellfish	Protein, fat, vitamin D, vitamin B12 and iodine	Meat, eggs

Living with the risk of an allergic reaction

Learning to live with the risk of an allergic reaction can be challenging, and for parents sending children out into the world, sometimes a little scary. You might worry about your child being offered food they can't be sure is safe, feeling left out when there are treats being offered, or even eating their allergen without realising.

It is, however, possible for you and your family to live a normal life, while minimising the risk of a serious allergic reaction. Ensure your child is educated about their allergy, and others caring for your child know what to do if an allergic reaction occurs.

The table below outlines the recommended daily intake of each food group for children at every age.

	Vegetables & legumes/beans	Fruit	Grain (cereal) foods, mostly wholegrain	Lean meat and poultry, fish, eggs, nuts and seeds, and legumes/beans	Milk, yoghurt, cheese and/or alternatives (mostly reduced fat)	Approx. number of additional serves from the five food groups or discretionary choices
These are the recommended average daily number of serves from each of the five food groups. Additional serves may be required for more active, taller or older children and adolescents.						
Toddlers						
1-2	2-3	½	4	1	1- 1½	–
Boys						
2-3	2½	1	4	1	1½	0-1
4-8	4½	1½	4	1½	2	0-2½
9-11	5	2	5	2½	2½	0-3
12-13	5½	2	6	2½	3½	0-3
14-18	5½	2	7	2½	3½	0-5
Girls						
2-3	2½	1	4	1	1½	0-1
4-8	4½	1½	4	1½	1½	0-1
9-11	5	2	4	2½	3	0-2½
12-13	5	2	5	2½	3½	0-2½
14-18	5	2	7	2½	3½	0-3

Preparing food at home

If your child is highly allergic to a particular food, they might suffer a reaction if their meal has been contaminated with ingredients from kitchen surfaces, cooking equipment or utensils.

You can decrease the risk of any reaction that is caused by cross-contamination by following these tips when preparing food.

- Use kitchen equipment that has been cleaned well using soap and water.
- Always wash hands with soap and water, and dry with a hand towel (paper or fabric) before touching other foods or switching between kitchen utensils. It's important to note that antibacterial gels will not remove food allergens.
- Store allergy-safe foods covered or in an airtight container away from other foods that may splatter or spill.
- Ensure any food items that have been removed from their packaging are clearly labelled.
- Thoroughly wash counters and tables with soap or household cleaner and water after preparing meals.
- Limit the sharing of food, drinks and utensils. Teach your child not to share these items when at school or with friends.
- Encourage hand and face washing for all family members after meals, especially when there are allergens present in the meal, to avoid skin exposure with hugs and kisses, and incidental touching.
- Take care with appliances and equipment that can lead to cross-contamination such as toasters, blenders, deep-fryers and barbecues. Keep one separate, or thoroughly clean items between use.
- If making separate meals, prepare the meals for your allergic child before preparing meals for the others in your family.

Limit the sharing of food, drinks and utensils. Teach your child not to share these items when at school or with friends.

Introducing solid foods

Introducing solids into your baby's diet can feel confronting if you're concerned about potential allergies, but research shows that starting common allergy-triggering foods within the first 12 months of a child's life can actually help to reduce their risk of developing an allergy to that particular food.

If you're concerned, always speak to your doctor, but when you're ready to introduce solids, these tips could help.

- Start feeding your baby solids at around six months of age (and not before four months).
- Introduce common allergens one at a time so, if there is a reaction, it's easy to identify the cause.
- If your child has any reaction to the food, immediately stop offering that food and see your doctor.
- These allergens should be introduced at around six months.
  - egg (well cooked)
  - peanut butter
  - cow's milk (only as a complementary food, not as the main milk drink)
  - tree nuts (prioritise those that are eaten regularly by the family)
  - soy
  - sesame
  - wheat
  - fish and other seafood (prioritise those that are eaten regularly by the family)
- Once you've introduced a food, keep giving it to your baby several times a week, unless they have a reaction. Trying it once or having it intermittently may not be enough to prevent an allergy from developing.
- Gradually build up enough variety to ensure your baby is eating a balanced diet, with foods from each food group eaten regularly.
- Giving your baby the same foods that you and the family are eating may encourage them to try new foods and be adventurous in their eating.

- Be mindful of your child's development and offer them food forms that are appropriate for their stage. For example, give them smooth nut butters spread on slices of bread, rather than whole nuts, while they're still learning to chew.
- Consider breastfeeding during the period that solid foods are first introduced to infants, from around six months. This may help reduce the risk of the infant developing allergies, although evidence for this is low.

Feeding toddlers and small children

Toddlers and small children can be fussy eaters, which can be frustrating if their diet is limited by allergies, but the following tips may help.

- Remember that it's your job to decide when food is offered and what type of food is offered, and it is then up to your child to decide if they are going to eat and how much.
- Try not to let your child fill up on milk, formula or fruit.
- Offer new foods in small amounts and with other foods your child already likes, but reassure them there is no pressure to eat them.
- Remember it's normal for your child's appetite to vary from meal to meal, and day to day.
- Try to eat with your child.
- Look at the texture, taste and colour of foods your child currently accepts eating, and then try new foods that are similar. For example, some children prefer to eat raw vegetables over cooked ones.
- Use imaginative talk and play, which can make trying new foods fun. For example, let's try licking the food like a lizard does, or nibbling on it just like a mouse.
- Get children involved in handling new

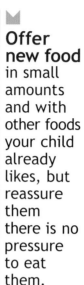

Offer new food in small amounts and with other foods your child already likes, but reassure them there is no pressure to eat them.

foods. For example, have them help with the grocery shopping, plant a vegetable garden, help with food preparation or serve the family meal.
- Stay calm and be patient. Keep your food acceptance expectations realistic, and don't give up!

Siblings

A common worry for families with children who have a food allergy is how to safely have the allergen in the house so others in the family can still have a normal diet. Some families choose to make all household meals and snacks free of the allergen, but this can be difficult, especially if you are managing multiple children with food allergies to different foods. It is also not the recommended approach.

Here are some suggestions that you may find helpful.

- Have a large container or a separate shelf in the pantry or fridge where the foods and snack items that are safe for the child with allergies can be stored.
- Have children eat at the same bench or table as much as possible, following the tips above on how to avoid cross-contamination.
- Allow children in the family without the food allergy to consume foods containing the allergen at a friend's place or at a time when a young sibling with allergies is at school or in childcare.
- Follow recipes that have substitutions for the common allergens and that would be suitable for the whole family to eat. We're sure that many of the recipes in this book will provide you with some inspiration!

Childcare and babysitters

If your child has a food allergy, it's important to only leave them with carers who know how to recognise an allergic

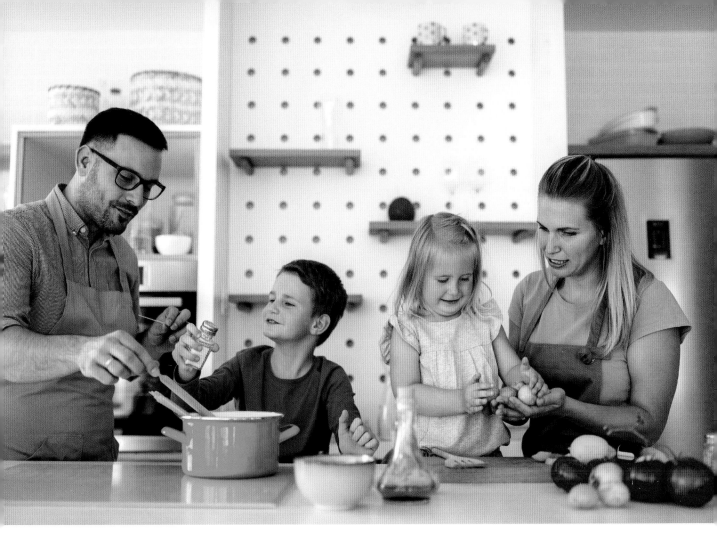

reaction and are able to administer any medication required. Before considering a childcare centre, check how many qualified staff they have, and what action plan they will implement if there is a medical emergency.

Babies weighing under 7.5kg cannot be treated with an EpiPen, and childcare staff are not qualified to administer adrenaline by any other means, so you may wish to speak to your doctor about options for childcare that will be able to keep a younger child safe.

Any babysitters you hire, and any family and friends who will be watching your child, should also be trained in how to recognise and manage an allergic reaction, including administering adrenaline if your child has been prescribed an adrenaline injector. It's important they also know to

Anyone watching your child should be trained in how to recognise and manage an allergic reaction, including giving adrenaline.

avoid eating or handling the allergen while they are caring for your child.

The Murdoch Children's Research Institute AllergyPal app can be a valuable support in helping to manage your child's allergy, and to keep your child safe when they are in someone else's care. This app also offers a convenient way to share your child's food allergy action plan with schools and childcare facilities. You can learn more about AllergyPal and download the app by scanning the QR code below.

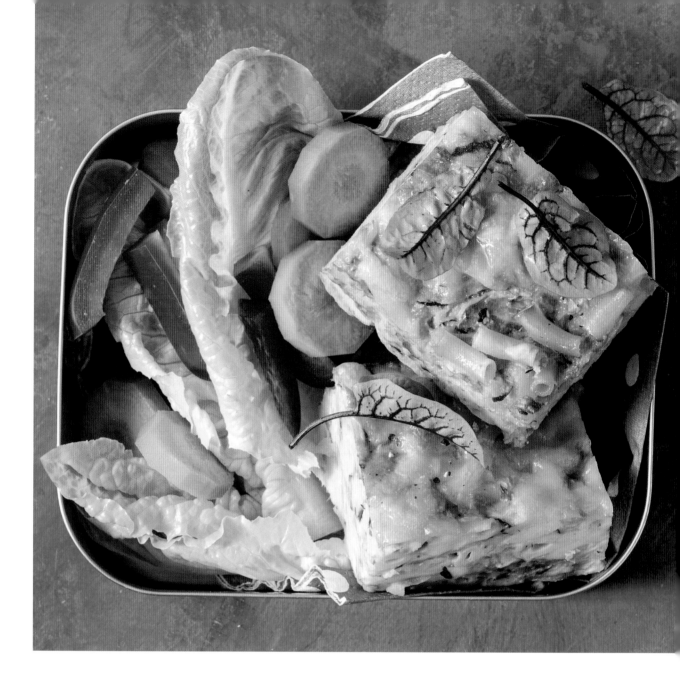

School

Starting school is an exciting yet potentially nerve-wracking time for children and parents, and for those also managing a food allergy, it can be particularly worrisome. For many parents, this will be the first time their children will be making some of their own decisions when it comes to food, so it's important those children with allergies are well prepared.

- Provide the school with an ASCIA food allergy (green) or anaphylaxis

Provide school with an ASCIA food allergy action plan and update it annually.

(red) action plan and update it annually (or any time it changes), so you can work together to keep your child safe.
- Provide your child's school with an adrenaline autoinjector (if prescribed), even though all Australian schools are required to have these made available, and staff trained to use them.
- Ensure your child never shares food with anyone, even if their school has a ban on their allergen being brought to school.

- Plan for when there are special events at school involving food; for example, when someone brings in treats for their birthday. Some parents leave a stash of treats with their child's teacher for such occasions, or the teacher may require all treats brought to class to be allergen free.
- Ensure your child feels comfortable speaking up in or out of class if they feel unwell.
- Label your child's lunchbox with "No [allergen]" to ensure others around them are aware. You can buy labels or write one yourself with a permanent marker.
- Carefully check the food labels of any processed snacks, or pack homemade food when possible.
- All children (whether they are allergic or not) should be encouraged to wash their hands before and after eating, to avoid inadvertent allergen contact.
- Teach your child to never assume a food is safe unless they have read and understood the label, or it's been packed at home for them. If they are unsure about a food, they should not eat that food.
- Talk to the tuckshop manager about their policy on allergens, and find out what foods are safe for your child to order. Check that these foods are not prepared in the same space as foods containing allergens. Some canteens will also put a photo of the child on their noticeboard along with their allergy details, so the child is not sold anything that could cause a reaction.
- If your child attends care outside school hours, talk to the manager about their policy on allergens, and ensure your child will be offered safe food options. Also, ensure there is always someone trained in how to recognise and manage an allergic reaction, including administering adrenaline, if required.

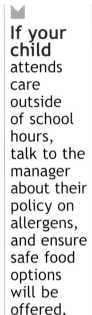

If your child attends care outside of school hours, talk to the manager about their policy on allergens, and ensure safe food options will be offered.

Eating out

With a little bit of planning, eating out can be a fun and social activity for you and your family. It can be difficult to know all ingredients in a dish, and many will have hidden and often unexpected ingredients, so it's important to ask questions to know for sure what is in each dish before you allow your child to eat anything. Here are some tips to get you by.

- Look online for a menu in advance, so you can plan ahead.
- Call ahead, if possible, and ask to speak to the chef. Ask their advice on the safest meals to eat, ask about every ingredient in the meals and double check they are not prepared in a way that could risk cross-contamination with other dishes in the kitchen. You can do this when you arrive, if you haven't planned ahead, but if the restaurant is busy it may be more difficult. Going at a less busy time can help.
- Always tell the wait staff and/or the chef about your child's allergy.
- Don't allow your child to share cutlery, straws or cups with others.
- Avoid seafood restaurants if your child is allergic to shellfish. Even if they don't order seafood, it can be difficult to avoid cross-contamination.
- Be careful of cross-contamination risks at Asian restaurants if your child has a severe peanut or tree nut allergy.
- Many Middle Eastern restaurants and patisseries can also pose cross-contamination risks, so be wary if your child has a severe sesame allergy.
- If fried food is ordered, check that it is not fried in the same oil as foods containing allergens.
- Avoid buffet restaurants where serving utensils can be shared and food accidentally mixed.
- Remember to also check the ingredients of garnishes and dressings, as these may contain allergens.

- Remember this rule of thumb: the fewer ingredients in a dish, the less chance there is for a hidden allergen to sneak through.
- Never assume that because something was safe at another restaurant, or even at the same restaurant, it will be safe everywhere and every time. Always ask.
- If you are unsure about what is in a dish, do not allow your child to eat it.
- Always carry snacks in case a situation arises where you can't find something for your child to safely eat.

Parties, sleepovers and special occasions

When going to a party or a friend's place, it's up to you to take charge of the situation so your child is kept safe. Your host may not have experience or understanding of how to manage allergies, or of what foods are safe or unsafe. Even if they assure you they are offering allergy-friendly food, it's okay to ask questions and double check ingredients and preparation arrangements in order to keep your child safe.

Here are a few tips to help out.

- Be clear about what foods your child can eat so that your host can plan appropriately.
- Ask for snacks containing allergens to be put on a higher table or kept separate from safe foods, to avoid any confusion.
- Teach your child to never take food from anyone else and, if they are younger, ask them to always check with you before eating anything.
- Ensure everyone knows about your child's allergy.
- Bring your own snacks so your child can eat those.
- Don't try new foods on special occasions like Christmas. Stick to what you know is safe and save experiments for times when you can be fully present and responsive.

Always ensure you have treats for your child so they don't feel left out or tempted to try a food that's unsafe due to hunger.

- If eating from a barbecue, have your child's food cooked first or on a piece of foil, and with separate utensils.
- Always ensure you have treats for your child so they don't feel left out or tempted to try a food that's unsafe due to hunger.
- Don't go anywhere without your child's medication.
- Learn where the local hospital is.

School camp

Going on school camp can be exciting for kids but nerve-wracking for parents concerned about a food allergy. Planning ahead and good communication with teachers and camp organisers is important to ensure it runs smoothly.

Scan the QR code below to go to Allergy & Anaphylaxis Australia for a full guide to Preparing for Camp with Food Allergies.

Teenagers

As your child gets older, they can start to take more responsibility for keeping themselves safe. This can be a relief, but also worrying, as you learn to let go and give your child more independence!

When your child begins high school, they have multiple classrooms and teachers, and it's important they have the confidence to communicate about their allergy clearly, and to manage their diet safely.

The high school years are also a time many children engage in risky behaviour. They need to understand the gravity of their allergy, and what to do if they do become unwell. Encourage your child to tell

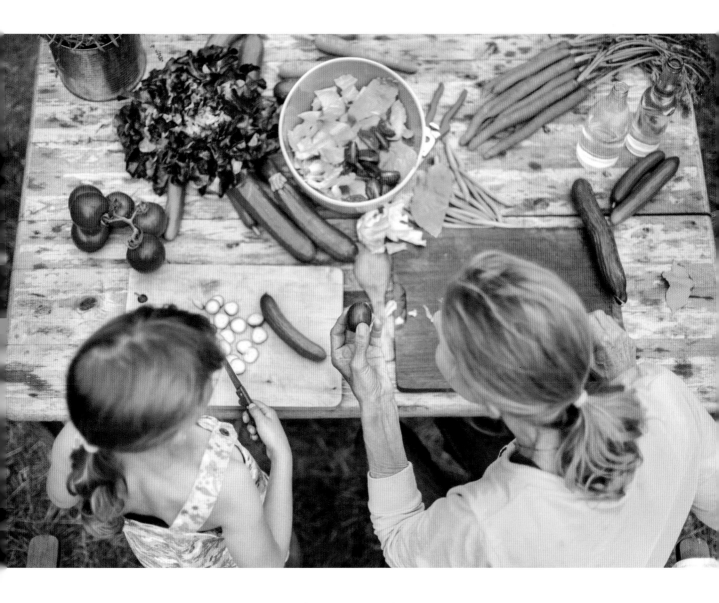

their friends about their allergy so they understand how to keep them safe.

As your child begins to make their own way in the world, these tips may help.

- Discuss with your teenager various ways they can make sure they have access to their allergy medication, especially at parties or when out with friends. This may include a sports belt that can be discreetly worn under clothing or a small bag. The most important thing to keep them safe in

Ask the school to inform all of your child's teachers of their allergy.

the event of accidental exposure to their allergen is having quick and ready access to medication.
- Print out a card that includes your child's name, allergies and medication required, and ask them to keep it with them.
- If they are willing to wear it, a medical information bracelet may be helpful.
- Ask the school to inform all of your child's teachers of their allergy, and work with the school to create a management plan in case of any reaction at school.

- Speak to the teacher in charge of the school year about the importance of avoiding allergens, especially if there is any cooking to be done at the school.

For comprehensive toolkits to help you manage your teen's allergy, scan the following QR codes.

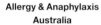

Allergy & Anaphylaxis Australia

Allergy 250K

It is essential you read all food labels carefully and you understand where allergens may be found.

Shopping tips

One of the most important skills for food allergy management is knowing how to read food product ingredient labels. It is essential you read all food labels carefully and you understand where allergens may be found in your grocery items.

In Australia, all food labels must contain a list of ingredients, including any allergens. This is governed by Food Standards Australia New Zealand (FSANZ). Ingredients are listed in descending order of weight, and the common allergens (peanut, tree nuts, milk, egg, fish, shellfish, wheat, sesame and soy) must all be declared, however small the amount.

This is an example of a food label, with allergens shown in bold and listed in 'contains' at the bottom.

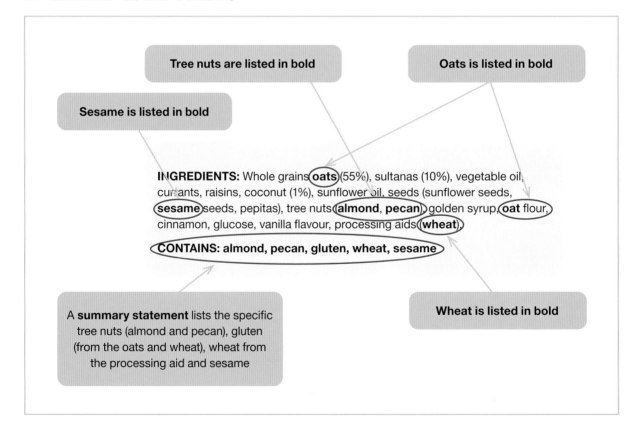

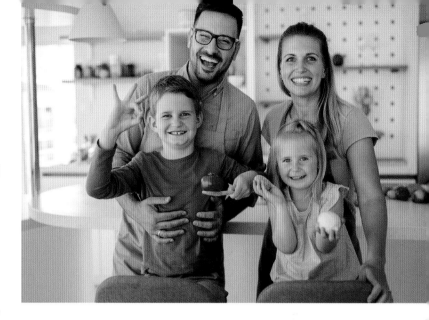

It is now also mandatory for allergens to be listed in "plain language"; that is, milk instead of casein or whey, and egg instead of albumin or livetin.

Some companies will also place a summary allergen statement at the end of the ingredient list.

Only proteins need to be avoided for food allergies. Some food components that are derived from potential allergenic foods are unlikely to contain the food protein because the allergen is removed or degraded during processing. For example, if the component is made up of just fats or sugars derived from the allergen.

Some examples of safe allergen derivatives include the following.

- Egg – egg lecithin, egg emulsifier
- Soy – soy emulsifier, soy lecithin
- Wheat – glucose, glucose syrup, dextrose, caramel colour and monosodium glutamate.

If you're unsure whether a derived ingredient is safe for your child, check with your doctor or allergist before allowing your child to eat it.

You may also see precautionary allergen statements on some packaged foods, such as "may contain traces of milk" or a disclaimer that the product is made in the same facility as products that contain an allergen.

These statements are currently voluntary, and there are no clear guidelines for companies on how and when to use them. The wording of the statements makes it difficult for parents and carers to determine the level of risk, and a product that does not contain the statement may in reality be no safer than a product that does. The chance of having a significant allergic reaction through contamination during food processing is low, however people with a food allergy should discuss what to do about food labels that contain precautionary allergen statements with their doctor or allergist.

Don't rely on labels that claim, 'Free from [allergen]'. Check ingredients yourself. It's better to be certain.

When you're learning to shop for your child with a food allergy, these tips on shopping safely may help.

- Allow extra time to ensure you are able to read all food labels carefully.
- Always read the labels on the food packaging, every time you purchase something, even if you've bought it before. Ingredients and the way foods are manufactured can change, and there is no requirement for a product to announce those changes.
- Keep in mind that your allergen may be known as something else, or hidden in another ingredient if the food comes from a country where the food labelling laws do not require listing the allergen in plain language. For example, milk may be listed as casein. Check for ingredients on food labels for your particular allergen as a starting point, but ensure you are well informed about any ingredients that could cause an allergic reaction.
- Don't rely on packaging labels that claim, 'Free from [allergen]'. Check the ingredients for yourself. It's always better to be certain.
- Mistakes can happen in translations on food products that have been imported from non-English-speaking countries, so be extra careful checking food labels translated from another language.

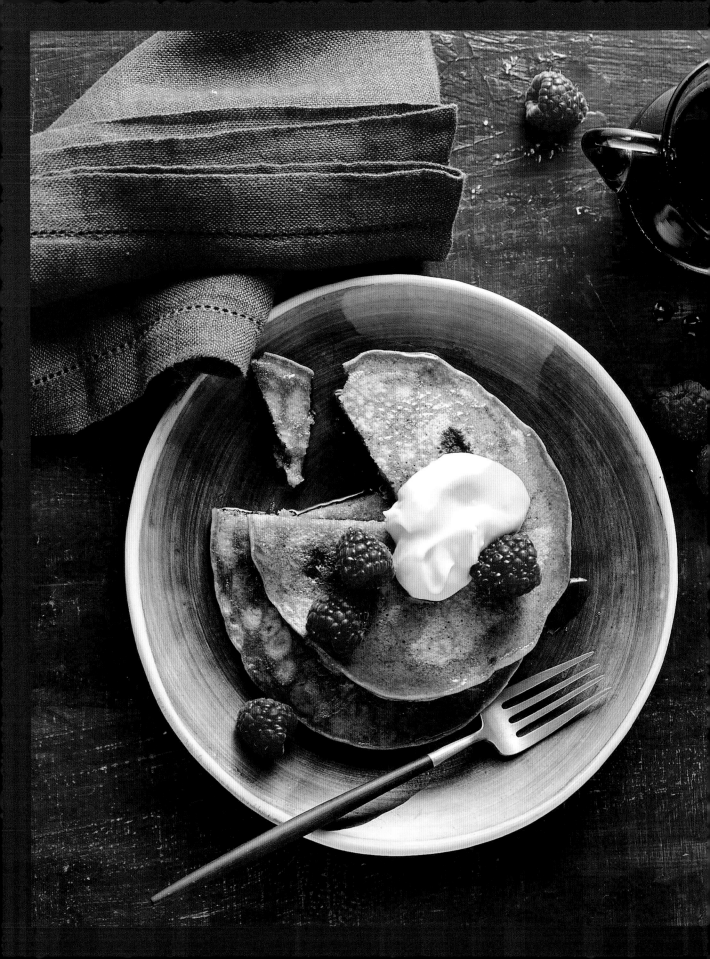

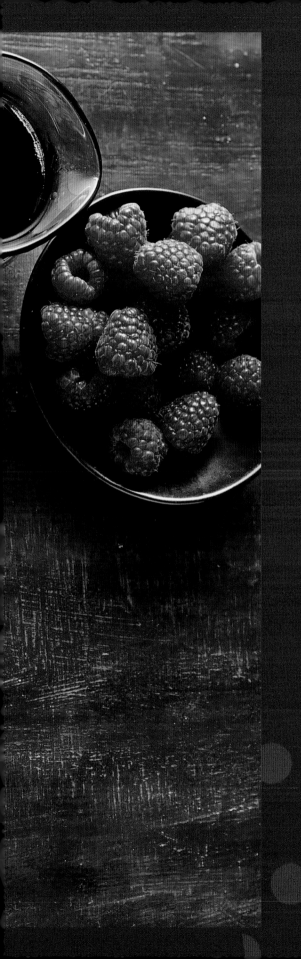

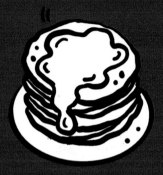

breakfast

Simple full-of-flavour dishes
that will set you up for
the rest of the day.

5-minute breakfast
BOWL

This nutrient powerhouse breakfast has a delicious sprinkling of crunchy nuts and seeds, and fresh fruit. As an added bonus, it takes just minutes to make.

serves 1   **prep** 5 mins

ingredients

1 small orange, peeled,
   pith removed
40g (¼ cup) quinoa, cooked
½ tsp ground cinnamon,
   plus extra, to serve
70g (½ cup) fresh blueberries
2 tsp finely chopped roasted
   unsalted almonds
3 tsp pepitas
80g (⅓ cup) natural yoghurt

1 Holding the orange over a bowl to catch the juice, use a sharp knife to remove the segments, cutting close to either side of the white membranes. Place segments in a separate bowl.

2 Add the quinoa and cinnamon to the bowl with the juice. Stir until well combined. Add orange segments, blueberries, almond and pepitas. Stir to combine. Top with the yoghurt and sprinkle with the extra cinnamon, to serve.

PER SERVE 12.2g protein, 11.8g fat (3.3g saturated fat), 33.8g carb, 8.7g dietary fibre, 312 Cals (1303kJ)

NUT FREE Simply omit the almonds. **DAIRY FREE** Swap the natural yoghurt for dairy-free coconut yoghurt. **BOOST** Add a handful of sultanas or chopped dates with the orange segments in step 2.

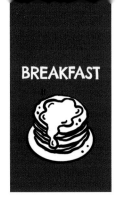
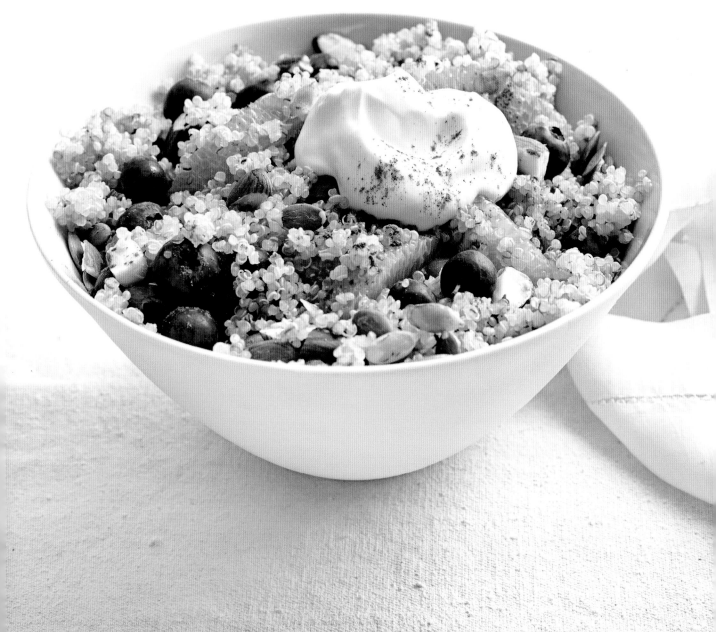

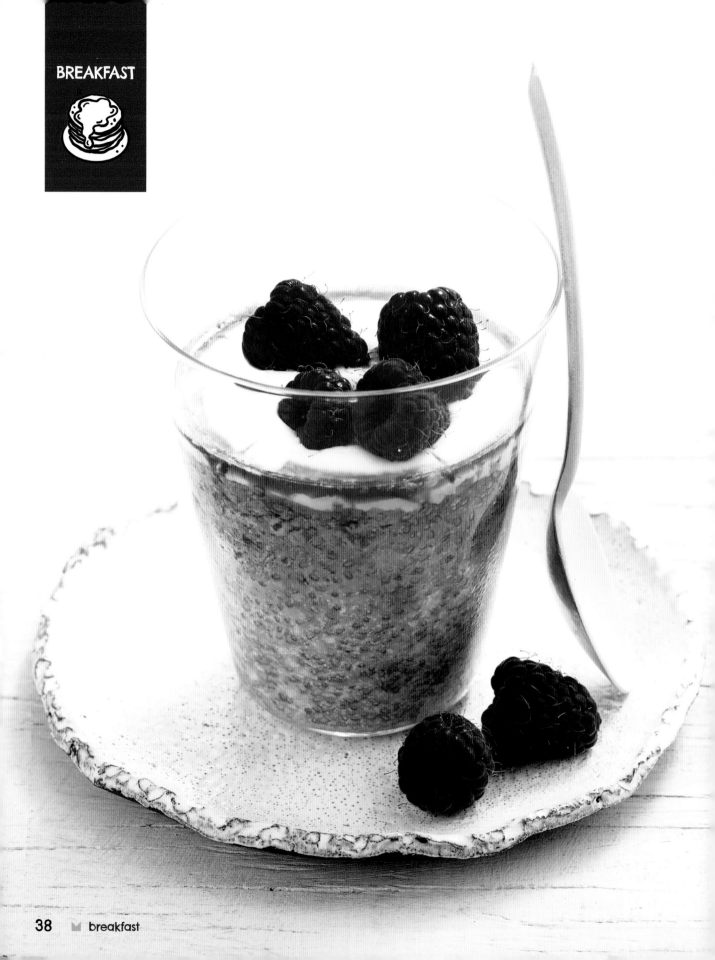

overnight berry + chia
QUINOA POTS

Kick-start your day with these colourful (and filling) make-ahead brekky pots brimming with tangy raspberries.

makes 2   **prep** 10 mins (+ overnight soaking)

ingredients

60g (½ cup) fresh raspberries or thawed frozen raspberries, plus extra 30g (¼ cup), to serve

40g (¼ cup) chia seeds

25g (¼ cup) quinoa flakes

2 tsp maple syrup

185ml (¾ cup) reduced-fat milk

90g (⅓ cup) natural yoghurt, to serve

1 Place the raspberries in a bowl and mash with a fork until fairly smooth. Add the chia seeds, quinoa, maple syrup and milk. Stir to combine. Divide mixture between two 250ml (1 cup) glasses.

2 Cover the glasses with plastic wrap and place in the fridge overnight to allow the flavours to develop and the seeds and quinoa to soften. Top pots with yoghurt and sprinkle with extra raspberries, to serve.

PER SERVE 11g protein, 10g fat (3g saturated fat), 22g carb, 11g dietary fibre, 250 Cals (1048kJ)

make it your way

DAIRY FREE Substitute the milk for a plant-based milk, and the natural yoghurt with any type of dairy-free yoghurt you desire. **MAKE AHEAD** Double or triple the recipe and make 4-6 pots to cater for more people or breakfast for a few days. Simply keep the glasses covered in the fridge for up to 3 days, until you're ready to serve.

pie maker cheesy
CORN FRITTERS

These easy vegetarian bites make a super satisfying family breakfast. Any leftovers can easily be popped into lunch boxes for a healthier snack at school or work. Just eat as is or warm in the microwave.

makes 12   **prep** 10 mins   **cook** 30 mins

ingredients

2 x 420g cans corn kernels, drained
55g (1 cup) finely grated cheddar
100g feta, crumbled
2 tbs chopped fresh chives, plus extra, to serve
75g (½ cup) gluten-free self-raising flour
Pinch of cayenne pepper (optional)
2 eggs
80ml (⅓ cup) milk
Light sour cream and sweet chilli sauce, to serve

1 Place the corn, cheddar, feta and chives in a large bowl. Use clean hands to mix until well combined. Add flour and cayenne, if using. Season with salt. Stir until well combined.

2 Make a well in the centre of the corn mixture. Whisk the eggs and milk in a jug. Pour the egg mixture into the well and fold in until just combined (do not over mix).

3 Preheat a pie maker. Lightly grease the pie maker holes with oil. Scoop a level ¼ cup of corn mixture into each hole. Close the lid and cook for 10 minutes or until cooked through (the tops will still be pale). Transfer to a wire rack. Repeat with the remaining mixture to make 12 fritters.

4 Season the fritters and serve warm or at room temperature topped with a dollop of sour cream, the sweet chilli sauce and a generous sprinkling of extra chives.

PER FRITTER 5.4g protein, 6.2g fat (3.4g saturated fat), 16g carb, 1.3g dietary fibre, 144 Cals (602kJ)

DAIRY FREE Use dairy-free cheddar and feta instead, and swap the milk and sour cream with your desired plant-based options.

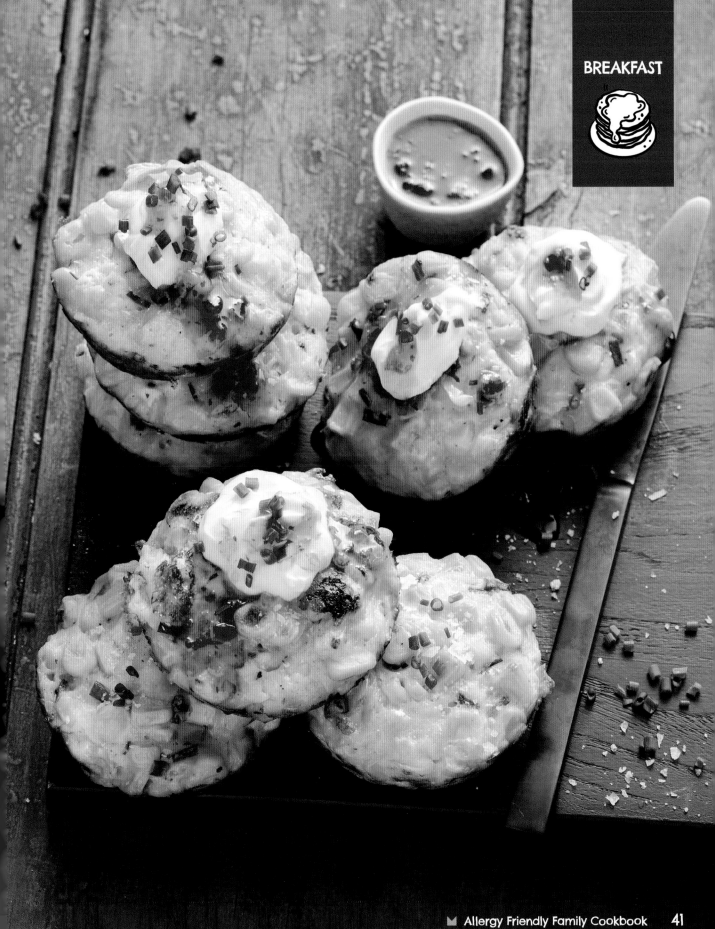

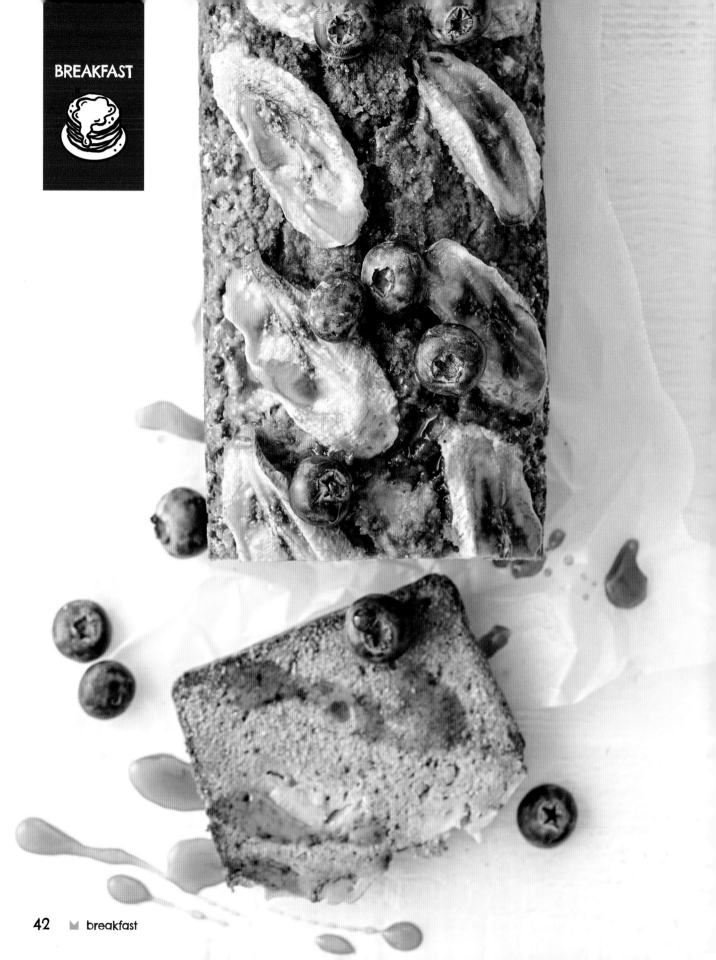

loaded gluten-free
BANANA BREAD

We call this our miracle banana bread! There's no refined sugar, dairy or gluten to be found, but it's light, moist and packed with sweet, sweet banana!

serves 12   **prep** 20 mins   **cook** 1 hour 10 mins

ingredients

180g (1 cup) brown rice flour
130g (1 cup) sweet potato flour
   or gluten-free plain flour
70g (½ cup) millet flour
1 tbs gluten-free baking powder
1 tsp ground cinnamon
½ tsp bicarbonate of soda
65g (⅓ cup) coconut sugar
   or rapadura sugar
400g (2-3 bananas) mashed
   banana, plus extra, sliced,
   to decorate
3 eggs, lightly whisked
185ml (¾ cup) almond milk
60ml (¼ cup) canola oil
Blueberries and maple syrup,
   to serve

1 Preheat oven to 170°C/150°C fan forced. Grease a 7cm-deep, 10.5 x 21cm (base size) loaf pan. Line the base and sides with baking paper, allowing the long sides to overhang.

2 Sift the flours, baking powder, cinnamon and bicarb into a large bowl. Stir in the sugar. Make a well in the centre. Add the banana, eggs, milk and oil to the well. Stir until just combined.

3 Spoon batter into prepared pan and smooth the surface. Decorate top with extra sliced banana. Bake for 1 hour 10 minutes or until a skewer inserted into the centre comes out clean. Cool in the pan.

4 Lift the banana bread from the pan. Cut into slices and serve with a scattering of blueberries and a drizzle of maple syrup.

PER SERVE 5g protein, 7g fat (1g saturated fat), 40g carb, 5g dietary fibre, 244 Cals (1020kJ)

make it your way

NUT FREE Swap almond milk with soy, oat or cow's milk, depending on your needs. BOOST Stir chopped dates into the batter in step 2.

super-quick quinoa
BIRCHER

For a healthy, low-calorie and gluten-free breakfast, try this deliciously easy quinoa bircher packed with fruit and seeds.

serves 2   **prep** 10 mins

ingredients
65g (⅔ cup) quinoa flakes
125g (½ cup) natural yoghurt
1 apple, coarsely grated
125ml (½ cup) soy milk
1 tbs sunflower seed kernels
2 tsp chia seeds
½ tsp ground cinnamon
½ cup fresh mixed berries (such as strawberries, raspberries and blueberries)

1 Combine the quinoa flakes, yoghurt, apple, milk, sunflower seed kernels, chia seeds and cinnamon in a bowl. Set aside for 5 minutes to soften. Top with the berries, to serve.

PER SERVE 12g protein, 9g fat (3g saturated fat), 41g carb, 7g dietary fibre, 312 Cals (1303kJ)

DAIRY FREE Swap the natural yoghurt for dairy-free coconut yoghurt. **SOY FREE** Swap the soy milk for cow's milk or rice milk.

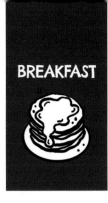

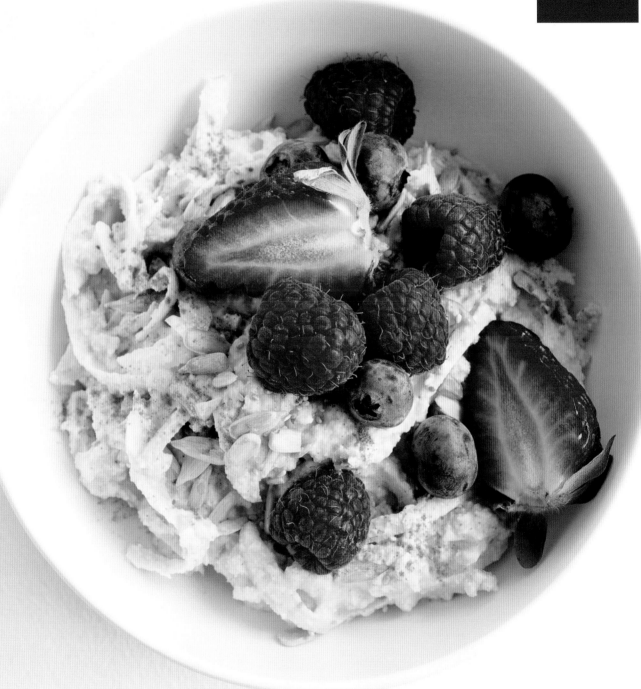

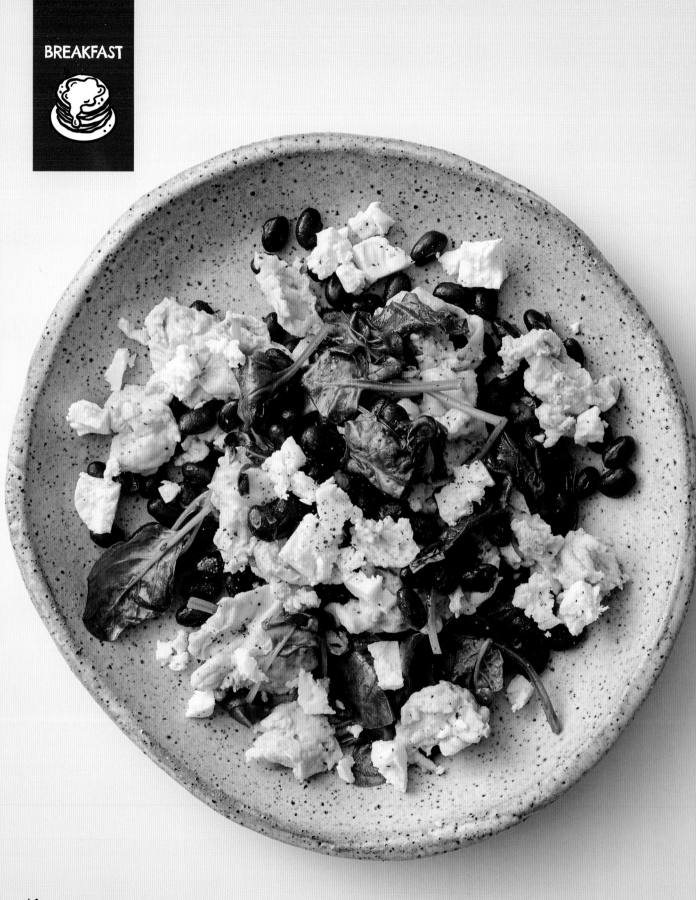

feta + black bean
SCRAMBLED EGGS

You only need 5 ingredients to whip up these good-for-you vegetarian scrambled eggs. They're on the table in just 10 minutes!

serves 1   **prep** 5 mins   **cook** 5 mins

ingredients
2 eggs
2 tbs unsweetened almond milk
125g can black beans, rinsed,
    drained
30g baby spinach
1 tbs crumbled Greek-style feta

1 Whisk the eggs and almond milk in a small bowl. Season. Heat a non-stick frying pan over medium heat. Lightly spray with olive oil.

2 Add the black beans and spinach to the pan. Cook, stirring, for 1-2 minutes or until the spinach is wilted. Transfer to a bowl.

3 Pour the egg mixture into the pan and cook, stirring gently with a wooden spoon, for 2 minutes or until the egg is just set. Stir through the spinach and bean mixture. Serve sprinkled with feta.

PER SERVE 20.7g protein, 15.4g fat (4.5g saturated fat), 11.1g carb, 5.6g dietary fibre, 280 Cals (1172kJ)

 DAIRY FREE Omit the Greek-style feta or swap it for vegan Greek feta. **NUT FREE** Use soy milk, or cow's milk (contains dairy).

quinoa coconut
PANCAKES

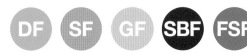

These fluffy golden pancakes might look like the real deal, but there's no gluten or dairy, so everyone gets to tuck into a 'stack' of the action.

serves 6 **prep** 10 mins **cook** 20 mins

ingredients

130g (1 cup) quinoa flour
60g (½ cup) coconut flour
55g (¼ cup) caster sugar
½ tsp bicarbonate of soda
½ tsp gluten-free baking powder
500ml (2 cups) almond milk
2 eggs
1 tsp vanilla bean paste
75g (½ cup) fresh raspberries, plus extra, to serve
20g (1 tbs) solid coconut oil, melted
280g (1 cup) dairy-free coconut yoghurt
125g (½ cup) pure maple syrup

1 Combine the flours, sugar, bicarb and baking powder in a bowl. Make a well. Whisk the milk, eggs and vanilla in a jug until combined. Pour into the well and stir to combine. Fold in the raspberries.

2 Heat a large non-stick frying pan over low heat. Brush with a little coconut oil. Cooking in 4 batches and brushing pan with oil between batches, pour ¼ cup batter into the pan for each pancake. Cook for 2 minutes or until golden underneath and bubbles form on the surface. Turn over and cook for 2-3 minutes or until golden underneath and cooked through. Transfer to a plate. Cover with foil to keep warm.

3 Serve the pancakes with yoghurt and extra raspberries, and drizzled generously with the maple syrup.

PER SERVE 9.2g protein, 17g fat (10.7g saturated fat), 55.7g carb, 4.7g dietary fibre, 427 Cals (1788kJ)

make it your way

NUT FREE Use any nut-free plant-based milk or cow's milk (contains dairy). **SWAP** Use thawed frozen raspberries in place of fresh.

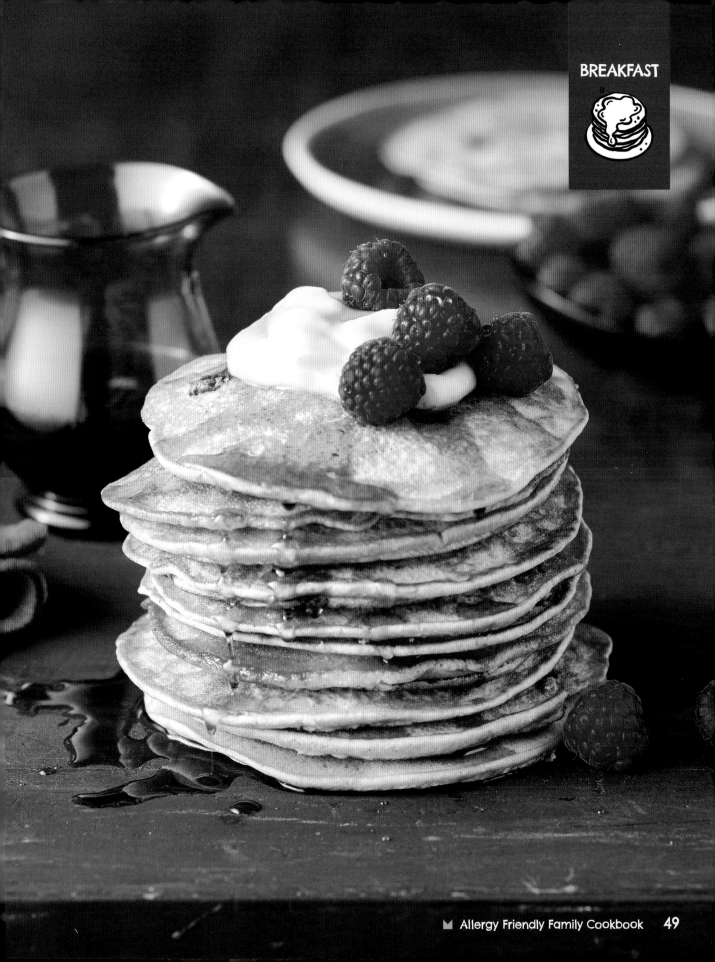

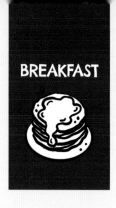

BREAKFAST

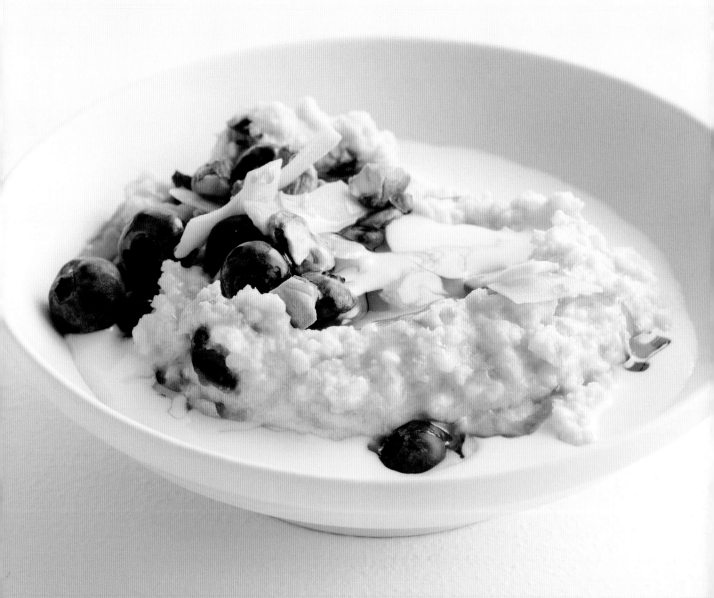

coconutty quinoa
PORRIDGE

This speedy brekky swaps rolled oats for low-GI and gluten-free quinoa for a super satisfying and warming start to your day. Top it with whatever fruit you have on hand.

serves 4   **prep** 5 mins   **cook** 5 mins

ingredients

230g (2 cups) quinoa flakes
250ml (1 cup) milk
3-4 fresh dates, pitted, chopped
125ml (½ cup) coconut milk,
   plus extra, to serve
125g punnet blueberries
40g (¼ cup) pistachios, chopped
Toasted coconut chips and
   maple syrup, to serve

1 Combine the quinoa flakes, milk and dates in a medium pan. Stir over medium-low heat for 3-4 minutes or until the mixture boils and thickens. Remove from the heat and stir in the coconut milk.

2 Spoon the porridge into serving bowls. Top with the blueberries and pistachio. To serve, sprinkle with coconut chips, and drizzle with extra coconut milk and maple syrup.

PER SERVE 13.1 protein, 23.2 fat (12.1 saturated fat), 67.4 carb, 6.9 dietary fibre, 531 Cals (2218kJ)

DAIRY FREE Replace the milk with almond, soy or rice milk, if you like.
NUT FREE Omit the pistachios or swap with extra fruit.

ultimate vegan
BREKKY WRAP

Packed with black beans and avocado, this quick and easy vegan breakfast wrap will fuel you for the day ahead. We love the added chilli hit, but you can use herbs instead if it's a little too hot to handle.

makes 1   **prep** 10 mins

ingredients

125g can black beans, rinsed,
   drained
Pinch of dried chilli flakes
   or mixed herbs
2 tsp fresh lemon juice
40g wholegrain wrap
20g baby spinach
1 roma tomato, sliced
¼ avocado, sliced
2 tbs fresh basil leaves
Lemon wedge, to serve
   (optional)

1 Place the black beans in a bowl and use a fork to coarsely mash. Combine the chilli and lemon juice in a jug and season.

2 Spread the bean mixture over the wrap. Top with the spinach, tomato, avocado and basil. Drizzle with the chilli mixture. Serve with the lemon wedge for squeezing, if you like.

PER SERVE 11.3g protein, 8.7g fat (1.9g saturated fat), 32.2g carb, 13.6g dietary fibre, 285 Cals (1190kJ)

GLUTEN & SOY FREE Swap the wholegrain wrap for a soy- and gluten-free wrap or tortilla of your choice. **TOAST IT** Fold the wrap in half and toast in a sandwich press until golden and crisp.

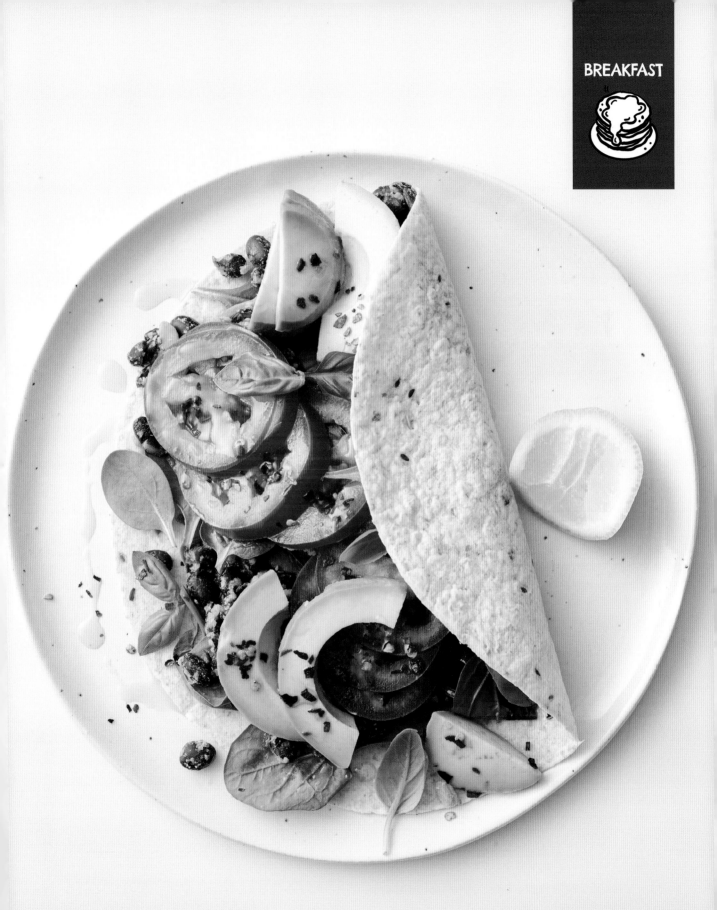

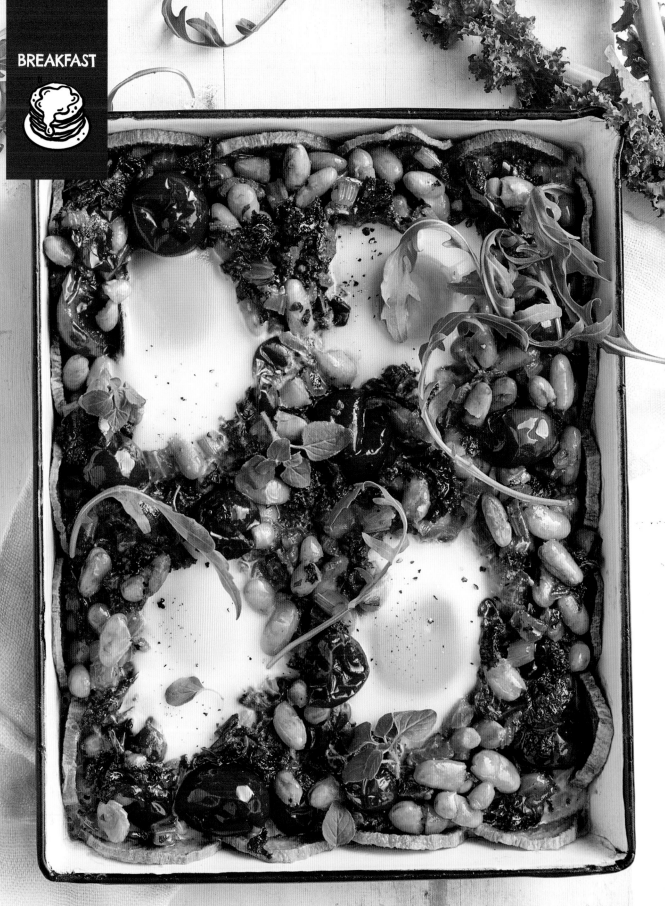

sweet potato, bean + kale
SHAKSHUKA

Abundant in fibre, this classic Middle Eastern dish is a hearty tomato-based breakfast the whole family will love.

serves 4   **prep** 15 mins   **cook** 40 mins

ingredients

500g sweet potato, peeled, cut into 5mm-thick slices.
1 tsp extra virgin olive oil
1 small red onion, finely chopped
2 celery sticks, finely chopped
2 garlic cloves, crushed
1 tbs chopped fresh oregano, plus extra sprigs, to serve
400g can cannellini beans, rinsed, drained
400g can cherry tomatoes
100g trimmed kale, torn into bite-sized pieces
4 eggs
Baby rocket and radicchio leaves, to serve

1 Preheat oven to 200°C/180°C fan forced. Spray a 16 x 26cm (base size) baking dish with olive oil. Place enough sweet potato slices, slightly overlapping, over base of prepared dish to cover. Cut remaining slices in half to create semi-circles. Use to line sides of the dish. Season. Spray with olive oil. Bake for 25 minutes or until golden and tender.

2 Meanwhile, heat the oil in a large saucepan over medium heat. Add the onion and celery. Cook, stirring, for 6-7 minutes or until softened. Add garlic and oregano. Cook, stirring, for 1 minute or until aromatic.

3 Add the beans and tomato to the pan. Bring to the boil. Reduce heat to low. Simmer, stirring occasionally, for 5 minutes or until thickened. Add the kale. Cook, stirring, for 2 minutes or until just wilted. Season.

4 Spoon bean mixture into sweet potato base. Make 4 shallow indents. Crack 1 egg into each indent. Bake for 15 minutes or until egg whites are just set but yolks are runny. Serve with rocket and radicchio leaves, and sprinkled with extra oregano.

PER SERVE 15g protein, 9g fat (2g saturated fat), 29g carb, 11g dietary fibre, 280 Cals (1170kJ)

EGG FREE Leave out the eggs, or swap for a sprinkling of crumbled dairy-free feta. Bake for 5 minutes before serving.

savoury tofu
SCRAMBLE

For a healthy allergy-friendly breakfast, skip the eggs and scramble some firm tofu with turmeric, spinach and cherry tomatoes. We guarantee you won't miss the eggs at all!

serves 1   **prep** 5 mins   **cook** 5 mins

ingredients
75g cherry tomatoes, halved

1 garlic clove, crushed

¼ tsp ground turmeric

100g firm tofu, crumbled

40g baby spinach

½ lime

½ x 45g wholegrain wrap,
    cut into wedges

1 Lightly spray a non-stick frying pan with olive oil and heat over medium-high heat. Add the tomato, garlic and turmeric. Cook, stirring, for 1 minute.

2 Add the tofu and spinach to the pan. Cook, stirring, for 2 minutes or until spinach has just wilted. Season. Transfer tofu scramble to a serving plate. Squeeze over the lime half. Serve with wrap wedges.

PER SERVE 15.4g protein, 6.8g fat (1.9g saturated fat), 20.2g carb, 5.9g dietary fibre, 193 Cals (808kJ)

make it your way

GLUTEN FREE Swap the wholegrain wrap for a gluten- and soy-free wrap or tortilla of your choice. **BOOST** Crumble a little dairy-free feta over the top of the scramble after plating.

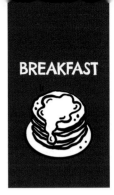

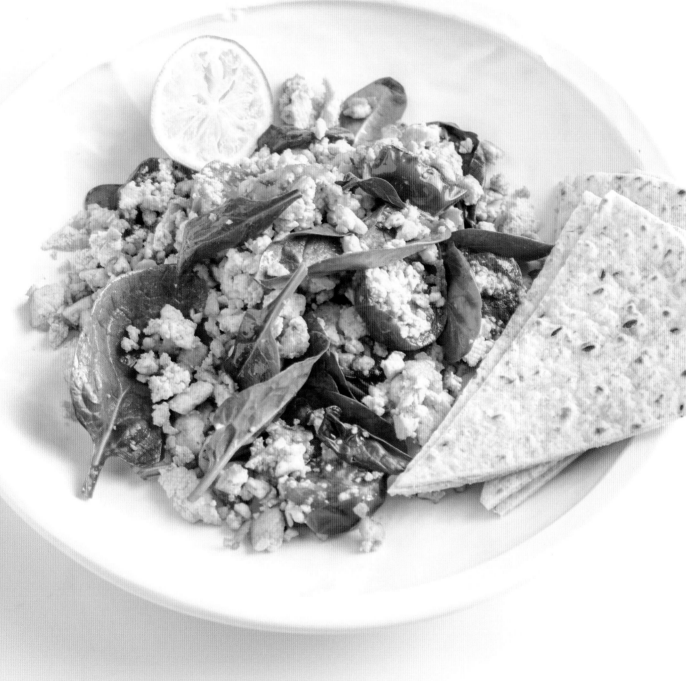

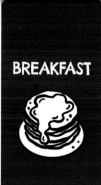

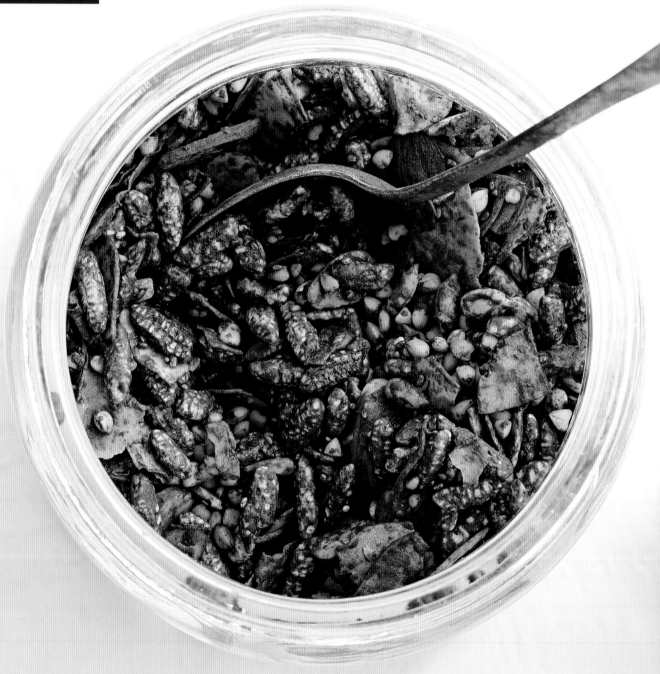

crunchy chocolate
GRANOLA

This gluten-free granola is a bit like that other popular chocolate puffed rice cereal the kids love, but it's so much better.

serves 4   **prep** 10 mins (+ cooling)   **cook** 25 mins

ingredients

50g (2½ cups) puffed rice
110g (2 cups) coconut chips
140g (1 cup) buckwheat
95 (1 cup) flaked almonds
80g (½ cup) sunflower
  seed kernels
2 tbs chia seeds
75g (⅓ cup) solid coconut oil
125g (⅓ cup) rice malt syrup
30g (¼ cup) cacao powder
Plant-based milk, to serve

1 Preheat oven to 150°C/130°C fan forced. Line 2 baking trays with baking paper. Combine the puffed rice, coconut chips, buckwheat, almonds, sunflower seed kernels and chia seeds in a bowl.

2 Place the coconut oil and rice malt syrup in a heatproof bowl. Microwave for 90 seconds. Whisk in the cacao powder. Add to the puffed rice mixture and stir to combine.

3 Evenly spread mixture over the prepared trays. Bake, stirring occasionally, for 25 minutes or until crisp. Cool. Serve with milk.

PER SERVE 9.7g protein, 27.5g fat (7g saturated fat), 32.4g carb, 6.8g dietary fibre, 426 Cals (1783kJ)

make it your way

NUT FREE Omit the almonds or replace them with 80g (½ cup) pepitas or 100g (1 cup) quinoa flakes, if you like. Use a nut-free milk.

marvellous mixed berry
PANCAKE BAKE

"Having a teenager with multiple food allergies, I've had years to experiment with new allergy-friendly recipes that are quick and easy. We love pancakes, and the great thing about this recipe is that I can bake one big tray to serve everyone at once." ~ *Lisa Gamble, Allergy Spot*

serves 8   **prep** 10 mins   **cook** 20 mins

ingredients

500g mixed berries (such as blueberries, raspberries and strawberries)
375g (2½ cups) self-raising flour
70g (⅓ cup) caster sugar
500ml (2 cups) oat milk
80ml (⅓ cup) vegetable oil
1 tsp vanilla extract
Pure icing sugar, to dust
Maple syrup, to serve

1 Preheat oven to 180°C/160°C fan forced. Grease a 3cm-deep, 23 x 33 cm (base size) baking dish.

2 Wash the berries and pat dry with paper towel. Hull and slice the strawberries, if using. Combine the flour and sugar in a bowl and make a well in the centre. Add the milk, oil and vanilla to the well. Whisk to combine.

3 Pour the batter into the prepared dish and smooth the surface. Gently press half the berries into the batter. Bake for 15-20 minutes or until springy to a gentle touch in the centre. Cool for 2 minutes.

4 Lightly dust pancake with icing sugar. Cut into 8 pieces and serve warm with the remaining berries and a drizzle of maple syrup.

PER SERVE 6.5g protein, 11.3g fat (1.2g saturated fat), 59.4g carb, 4.7g dietary fibre, 373 Cals (1560kJ)

GLUTEN FREE Use gluten-free self-raising flour. Note, the pancake may not rise as much and will have a denser texture. The cooking time may also vary slightly. Use gluten-free oat milk or another nut-free and dairy-free plant-based milk.

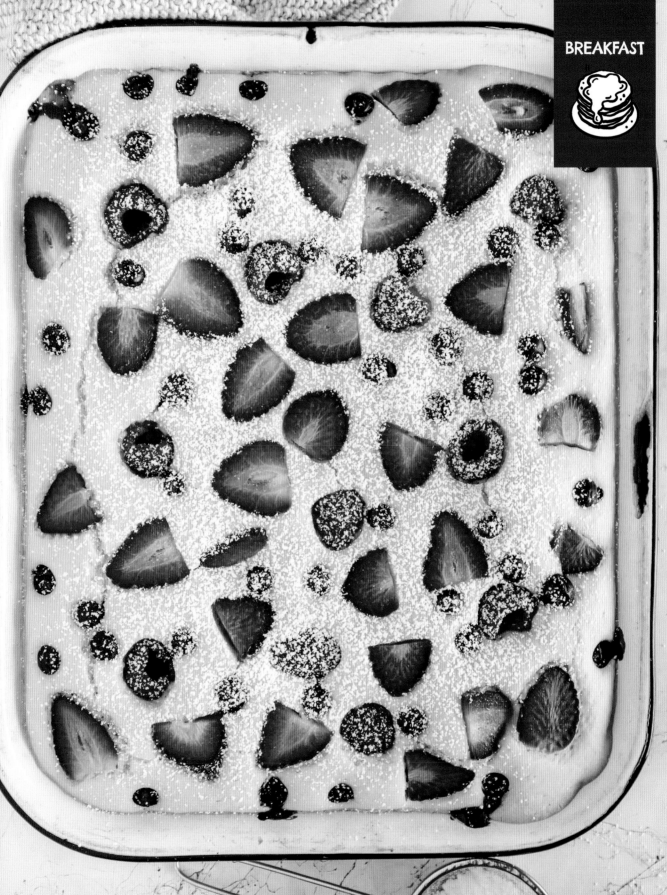

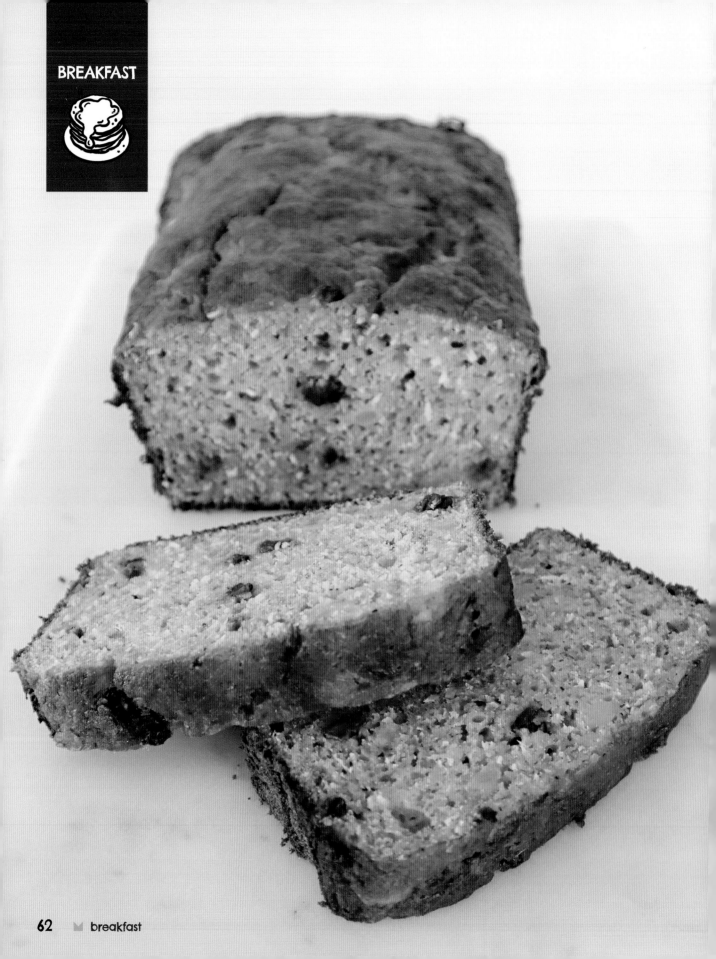

community recipe
spiced banana
BREAD

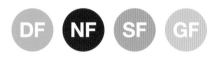

"I wanted a recipe to cater to the multiple allergies and food intolerances in our household. I adapted this recipe from a number I'd seen. The addition of apple sauce enriches the flavour and helps to take away the usual dryness and crumbliness of gluten-free recipes without them becoming too moist." ~ *Kat Meldrum*

serves 10   **prep** 15 mins (+ cooling)   **cook** 40 mins

ingredients

3 large bananas, mashed
60ml (¼ cup) vegetable oil
2 eggs, lightly whisked
2 tbs apple puree
2 tsp finely grated ginger
100g (½ cup) raw caster sugar
45g (½ cup) desiccated coconut
150g (1 cup) gluten-free
    plain flour
2 tsp gluten-free baking powder
1 tsp ground turmeric
1 tsp ground cinnamon
1 tsp ground cardamom
½ tsp ground black pepper
    (optional)
90g (½ cup) sultanas

1 Preheat oven to 200°C/180°C fan forced. Grease a 10 x 20cm (base size) loaf pan. Line the base and sides with baking paper, extending paper above the 2 long sides.

2 Combine the banana, oil, egg, apple puree and ginger in a large bowl. Stir in the sugar and coconut until combined.

3 Sift the flour, baking powder and spices into the bowl and stir to combine. Fold through the sultanas. Transfer the batter to the prepared pan and smooth the surface.

4 Bake for 40 minutes or until golden and a skewer inserted into the centre comes out clean. Cool in the pan for 10 minutes before transferring to a wire rack to cool completely.

PER SERVE 3g protein, 9.7g fat (3.5g saturated fat), 34.9g carb, 2.3g dietary fibre, 241 Cals (1008kJ)

make it your way

EGG FREE Swap eggs with the equivalent amount of egg replacer.
FREEZE Wrap slices in plastic wrap and freeze for up to 2 months.

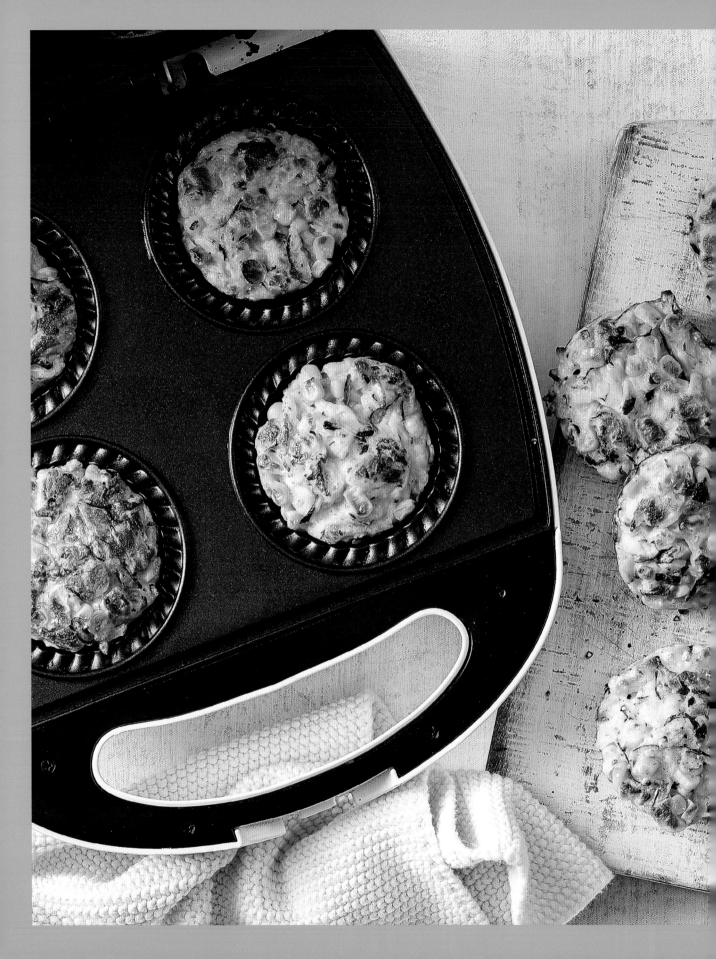

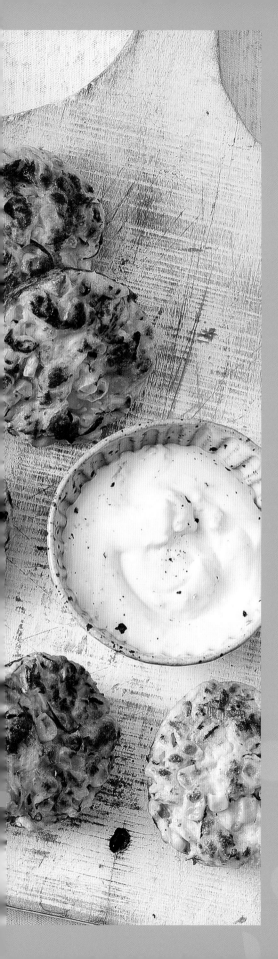

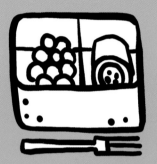

lunch + snacks

Plates that will make your (mid)day, plus snacks to satisfy cravings and the 3pm slump.

rice paper rolls with
CHICKEN

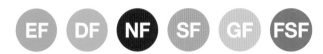

Coconut-poached chicken bundled up with fresh salad vegetables and a tangy chilli sauce — what's not to love?!

serves 4   prep 30 mins (+ standing)   cook 20 mins

ingredients

400ml can coconut milk

2 chicken breast fillets

100g dried vermicelli rice noodles

1 small red capsicum, thinly sliced

100g snow peas, trimmed, thinly sliced

1 small carrot, peeled, coarsely grated

100g (1½ cups) bean sprouts, trimmed

160g (½ cup) sweet chilli sauce

2 tbs fresh lime juice

12 large dried rice paper rounds

12 large fresh mint leaves

12 fresh coriander sprigs

1 Place the coconut milk, 375ml (1½ cups) water and chicken in a saucepan. Bring to a simmer over medium heat. Reduce heat to low. Cook, uncovered, for 20 minutes or until chicken is cooked through. Transfer chicken to a board to cool slightly, then thinly slice.

2 Meanwhile, cook noodles following packet directions. Drain. Refresh under cold water. Drain. Place in a large bowl. Use kitchen scissors to coarsely cut noodles in the bowl. Add capsicum, snow peas, carrot and sprouts. Season. Toss to combine.

3 Combine sweet chilli sauce and lime juice in a small bowl. Half-fill a shallow dish with warm water. One at a time, dip a rice paper round into the water. Place on a board. Stand for 20-30 seconds or until soft. Place a little chicken, 1 mint leaf and 1 coriander sprig along the centre. Top with 2 tbs noodle mixture. Fold in rice paper edges, then roll to enclose filling. Place on a serving plate. Cover with a damp tea towel to prevent drying. Serve rice paper rolls with the dipping sauce.

PER SERVE 35.9g protein, 5.3g fat (2.4g saturated fat), 74.5g carb, 5.4g dietary fibre, 500 Cals (2091kJ)

make it your way

SOY FREE Replace the bean sprouts with snow pea sprouts.
VEGETARIAN Omit the chicken fillets. Begin the recipe at Step 2.

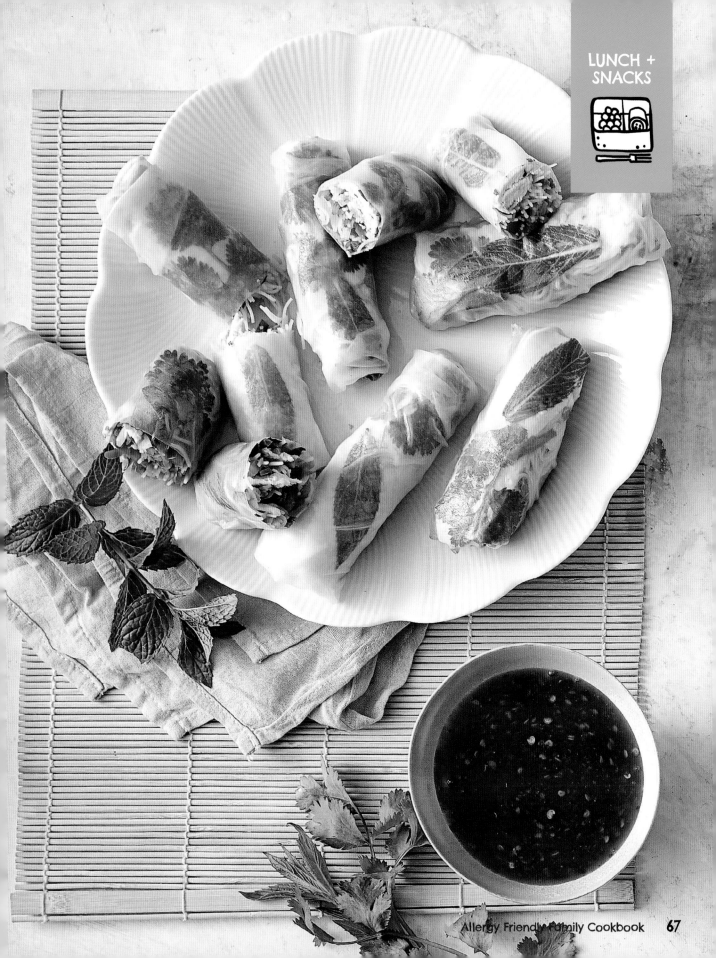

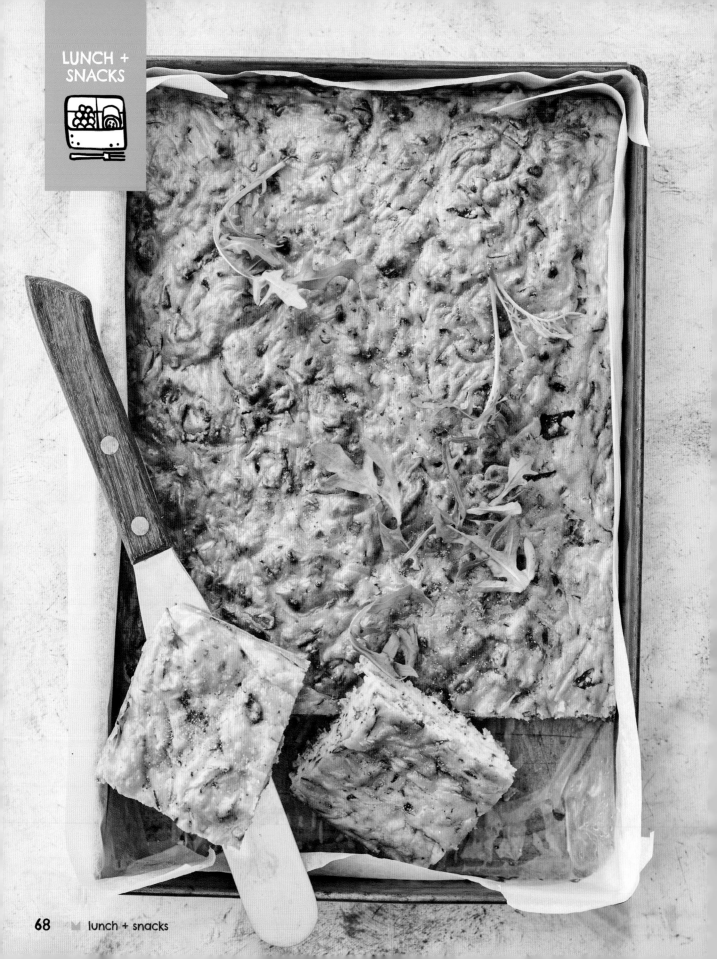

wheat-free
ZUCCHINI SLICE

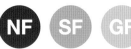

NF **SF** **GF** **SBF** **FSF**

Here's our super-tasty gluten-free version of the classic zucchini slice. Pop it in the oven for a veg-packed healthier lunch.

makes 12   prep 15 mins (+ cooling)   cook 40 mins

ingredients

2 tsp extra virgin olive oil,
   plus an extra 60ml (¼ cup)
150g smoked gluten-free bacon,
   finely chopped
1 brown onion, finely chopped
5 eggs
100g (⅔ cup) gluten-free
   self-raising flour
1 tsp gluten-free baking powder
380g (about 2) zucchini,
   coarsely grated, excess
   moisture squeezed out
80g cheddar, coarsely grated
Rocket leaves or salad leaves,
   to serve

1 Preheat oven to 200°C/180°C fan forced. Grease a 20 x 30cm (base size) slice pan and line with baking paper.

2 Heat the oil in a small frying pan over high heat. Add the bacon and onion. Cook, stirring, for 7 minutes or until bacon is crisp and onion is softened. Set aside to cool slightly.

3 Use a fork to whisk the eggs in a large bowl until combined. Add the flour and baking powder and stir until smooth. Add the zucchini, cheese, bacon mixture and extra oil. Stir to combine. Pour mixture into the prepared pan.

4 Bake slice for 30 minutes or golden and set. Cool for 10 minutes. Cut the slice into 12 pieces. Serve with rocket or salad leaves.

PER SERVE 9.1g protein, 6.1g fat (2.9g saturated fat), 8.3g carb, 0.9g dietary fibre, 133 Cals (554kJ)

make it your way
DAIRY FREE Substitute the cheddar for dairy-free cheese.
BOOST Serve with a hearty salad for a more filling meal.

mexican polenta
MUFFINS

Whip up a batch of these gluten-free low-carb muffins. Packed with vegies, fibre and healthy fats, they'll keep you full all afternoon long.

makes 9   prep 20 mins   cook 25 mins

ingredients

150g (1 cup) gluten-free
  self-raising flour
2 tsp gluten-free baking powder
170g (1 cup) fine polenta
1 long fresh red chilli, deseeded,
  finely chopped
4 green shallots, finely chopped
285g (1½ cups) fresh corn
  kernels
200g roasted red capsicum
  (not in oil), coarsely chopped
2 eggs
2 tbs extra virgin olive oil
125ml (½ cup) unsweetened
  almond milk
70g feta, crumbled
Avocado, mashed, to serve

1 Preheat oven to 190°C/170°C fan forced. Line nine 185ml (¾ cup) muffin pans with paper cases. Sift the flour and baking powder into a large bowl. Stir in the polenta, chilli, shallot, 185g (1 cup) corn kernels, and three-quarters of the capsicum. Combine the remaining corn and capsicum in a small bowl and set aside.

2 Whisk the eggs, oil and milk in a jug. Add to the polenta mixture and stir until just combined. Stir through the feta.

3 Divide mixture among the paper cases. Bake for 20-25 minutes or until muffins are golden and a skewer inserted into the centres comes out clean. Serve warm or at room temperature topped with mashed avocado and sprinkled with reserved corn and capsicum.

PER SERVE 6.1g protein, 7.9g fat (2.2g saturated fat), 32.3g carb, 2.3g dietary fibre, 229 Cals (957kJ)

make it your way

DAIRY FREE Swap the feta for dairy-free feta. NUT FREE Substitute the almond milk for any nut-free plant-based milk you desire.

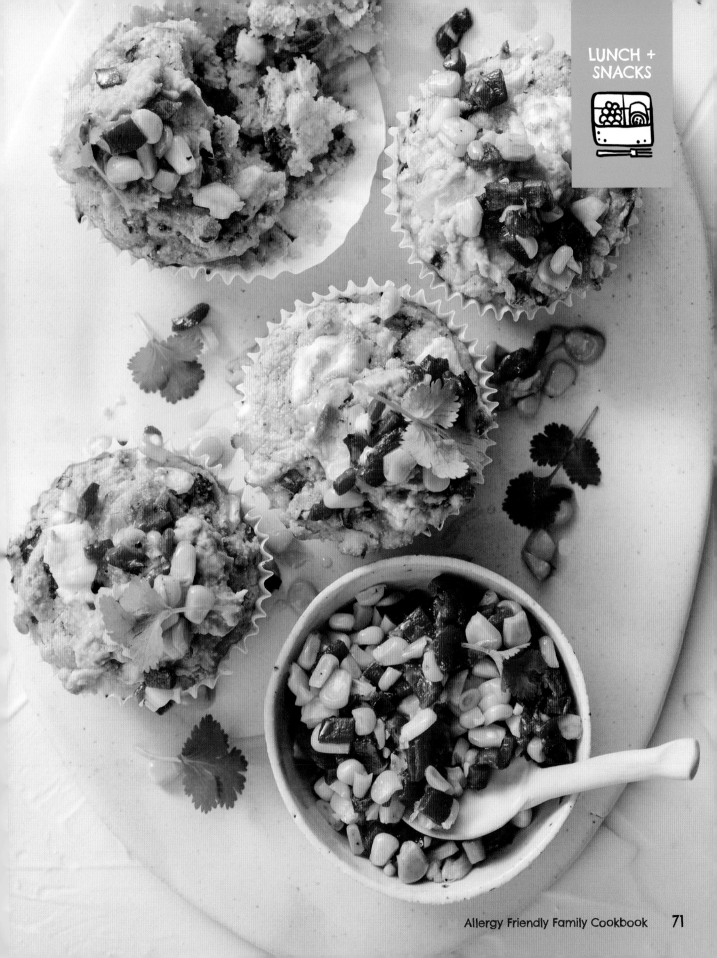

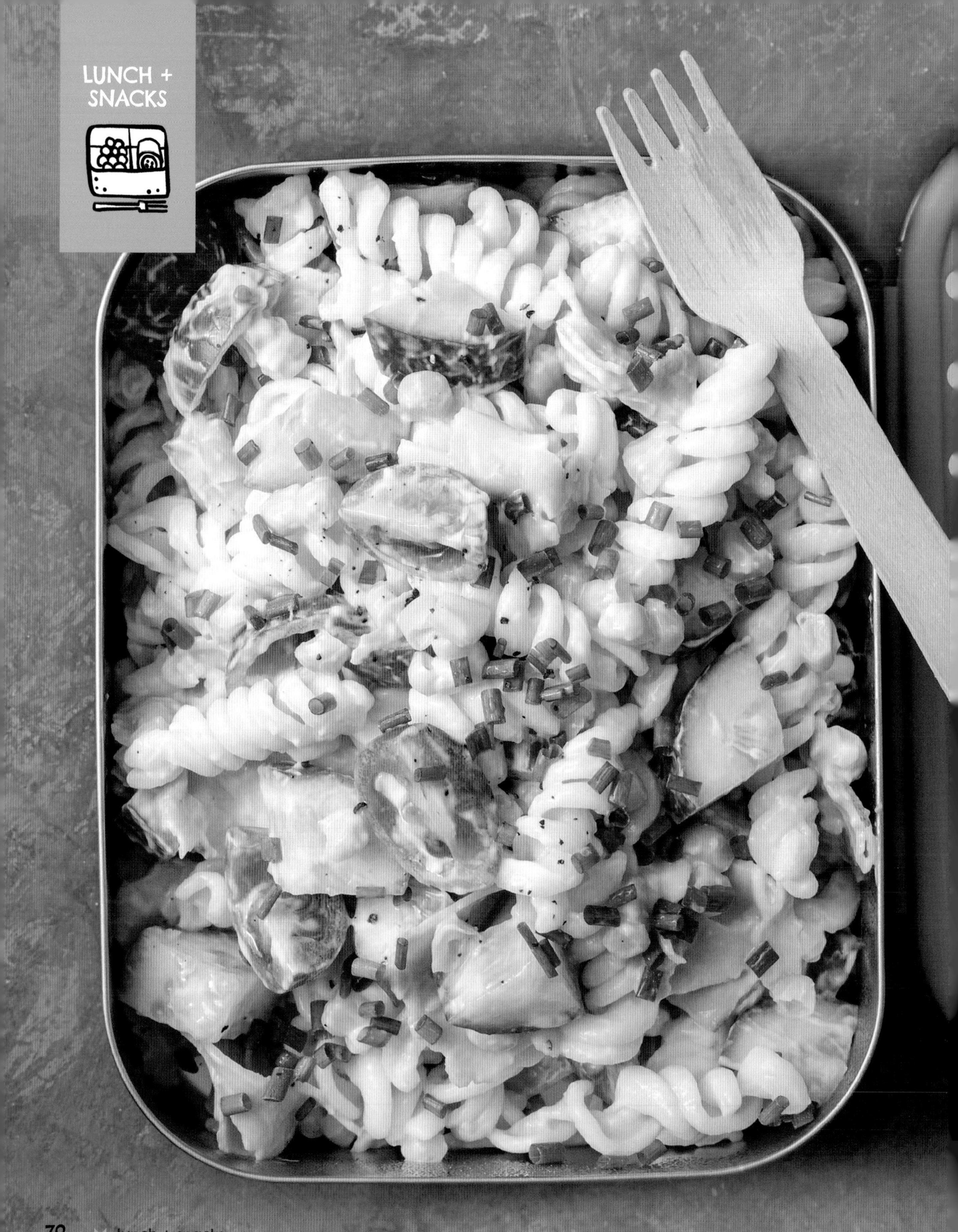

ham + corn
PASTA SALAD

Perfect for the lunch box, this creamy pasta salad is high in fibre and will keep the kids going till dinnertime. It's also ready in just 20 minutes.

serves 4   prep 10 mins   cook 10 mins

ingredients

180g (2 cups) dried fusilli pasta
125g (½ cup) reduced-fat
    whole-egg mayonnaise
1 tbs fresh lemon juice
300g can corn kernels,
    drained, rinsed
125g cherry tomatoes,
    quartered
1 Lebanese cucumber,
    quartered, chopped
100g shaved reduced-fat ham,
    coarsely chopped
Finely chopped fresh chives,
    to serve

1 Cook the pasta in salted boiling water following packet directions or until al dente. Drain. Refresh under cold water. Drain well.

2 Meanwhile, combine the mayonnaise and lemon juice in a large bowl. Stir in the cooled pasta until well combined.

3 Add the corn, tomato, cucumber and ham to the pasta mixture. Season and toss to combine. Serve sprinkled with chives.

PER SERVE 13.4 protein, 25.7 fat (3.6 saturated fat), 50.9 carb, 4.9 dietary fibre, 501 Cals (2098kJ)

make it your way

EGG FREE Swap the whole-egg mayonnaise for vegan mayonnaise.
GLUTEN FREE Use gluten-free pasta instead of regular pasta.

kale + cannellini bean
FALAFELS

These healthy homemade falafels are cooked in the oven so they're crispy and crunchy, but good for you, too. Plate and serve, or wrap it all up for a delicious lunch.

serves 4   prep 20 mins   cook 40 mins

ingredients

2 tsp extra virgin olive oil
1 brown onion, finely chopped
2 garlic cloves, crushed
2 tsp ground cumin
1 tsp ground coriander
125g trimmed kale, chopped
35g (⅓ cup) quinoa flakes
2 x 400g cans cannellini beans, rinsed, drained
½ cup fresh herbs (such as mint, parsley or basil), chopped
200g grape tomatoes, halved
100g rocket or baby spinach
130g (½ cup) hummus

1 Grease a baking tray and line with baking paper. Heat half the oil in a large non-stick frying pan over medium heat. Add the onion and cook, stirring, for 5 minutes or until softened. Add the garlic, cumin and coriander. Cook, stirring, for 1 minute or until aromatic. Add the kale and cook, stirring, for 3-4 minutes or until wilted. Set aside to cool. Transfer to a food processor.

2 Preheat oven to 190°C/170°C fan forced. Add the quinoa flakes, beans and half the herbs to the food processor. Process until combined and smooth. Season. Transfer mixture to a bowl.

3 Roll tablespoonfuls of the bean mixture into balls and place on the prepared tray. Flatten slightly with a fork. Lightly spray with oil. Bake, turning once, for 30-35 minutes or until golden.

4 Combine the tomato, remaining herbs and oil in a bowl. Season. Serve falafels with tomato salad, rocket or spinach, and hummus.

PER SERVE 14g protein, 10g fat (2g saturated fat), 27g carb, 15g dietary fibre, 283 Cals (1186kJ)

make it your way

SESAME FREE Omit the hummus or swap it for tahini-free garlic dip.
WRAP IT Place all components in a gluten-free wrap to eat on the go.

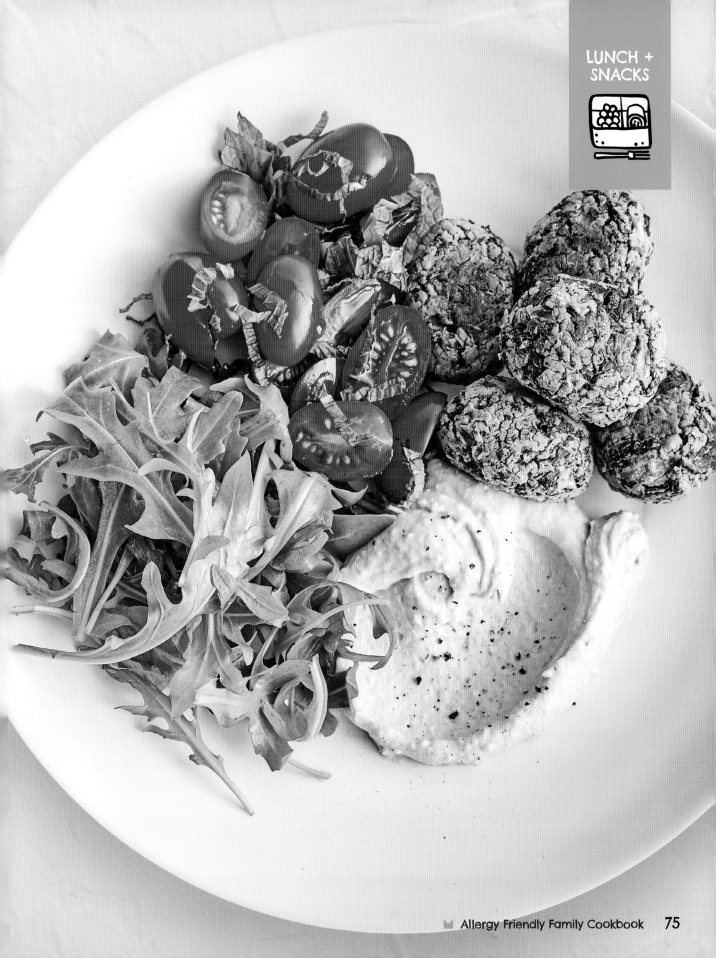

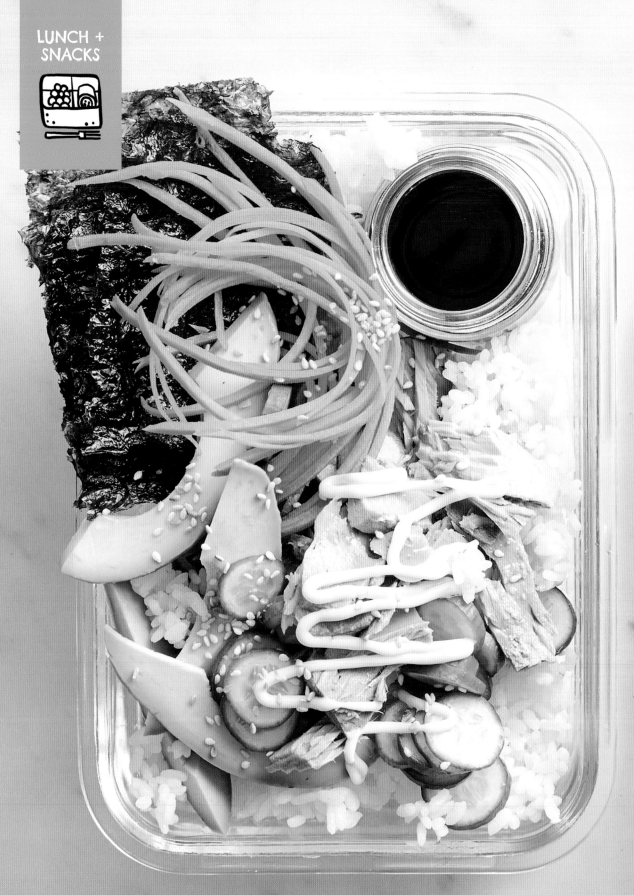

tuna + avocado
SUSHI SALAD

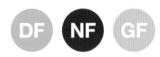

This sushi-style box is a sure-fire crowd pleaser. Make up a batch of the sushi rice and let your kids help choose the toppings.

serves 4   prep 10 mins   cook 15 mins

ingredients

325g (1½ cups) sushi rice
80ml (⅓ cup) sushi seasoning
1 large carrot, peeled
4 qukes (baby cucumbers)
2 small avocados, sliced
185g can tuna in olive oil, drained, flaked
1 tbs Kewpie mayonnaise
2 tsp sesame seeds, toasted
80ml (⅓ cup) salt-reduced tamari sauce
Roasted nori, to serve

1 Cook the rice following packet directions. Spread over a large baking tray. Drizzle with sushi seasoning. Toss to combine. Set aside to cool.

2 Meanwhile, use a julienne peeler or sharp knife to cut the carrot into long thin strips. Thinly slice the qukes.

3 Divide the rice among 4 lunch boxes. Top each with one-quarter of the cucumber, avocado, carrot and tuna. Drizzle mayonnaise over the tuna. Sprinkle with sesame seeds. Cover and place in the fridge until required. Divide tamari sauce among 4 small containers. Serve salad with the tamari sauce and roasted nori.

PER SERVE 16.1g protein, 21.1g fat (3.9g saturated fat), 74.1g carb, 5g dietary fibre, 565 Cals (2363kJ)

make it your way

EGG FREE Substitute the Kewpie mayo for vegan mayonnaise.
SESAME FREE Simply leave out the sesame seeds altogether.

pie maker zucchini
FRITTERS

We've made this family favourite even easier by adapting the recipe to suit a pie maker. These will go quickly, so think about making a double batch to go around.

makes 12   prep 20 mins   cook 40 mins

ingredients

1 tsp olive oil
3 green shallots, trimmed, thinly sliced
2 garlic cloves, crushed
500g (about 3) zucchini, coarsely grated
250g haloumi, coarsely grated
400g can corn kernels, rinsed, drained
100g (⅔ cup) self-raising flour
2 eggs, lightly whisked

lemon dipping sauce

125g (½ cup) mayonnaise
65g (¼ cup) light sour cream
1 tbs fresh lemon juice

1 Heat the oil in a small frying pan over medium heat. Add shallot and garlic. Cook, stirring, for 3 minutes until soft. Transfer to a large bowl.

2 Use hands to squeeze excess liquid from the zucchini then place in a large bowl. Add the haloumi, corn, flour and egg. Season with pepper and stir to combine.

3 Preheat a pie maker. Place ⅓ cup mixture in each hole. Spray lightly with oil. Close the lid and cook for 12 minutes or until golden and set. Lift out fritters and transfer to a wire rack. Repeat with the remaining mixture to make 12 fritters in total.

4 To make the dipping sauce, place the mayo, sour cream and lemon juice in a small bowl. Stir to combine. Serve fritters with dipping sauce.

PER SERVE 22.9g protein, 46.2g fat (13.6g saturated fat), 34g carb, 4g dietary fibre, 651 Cals (2723kJ)

make it your way

DAIRY FREE Swap the haloumi for dairy-free cheddar or pizza cheese. Instead of our dipping sauce, try making a sauce using 180g (¾ cup) sweet chilli sauce combined with 1 tbs fresh lemon juice.

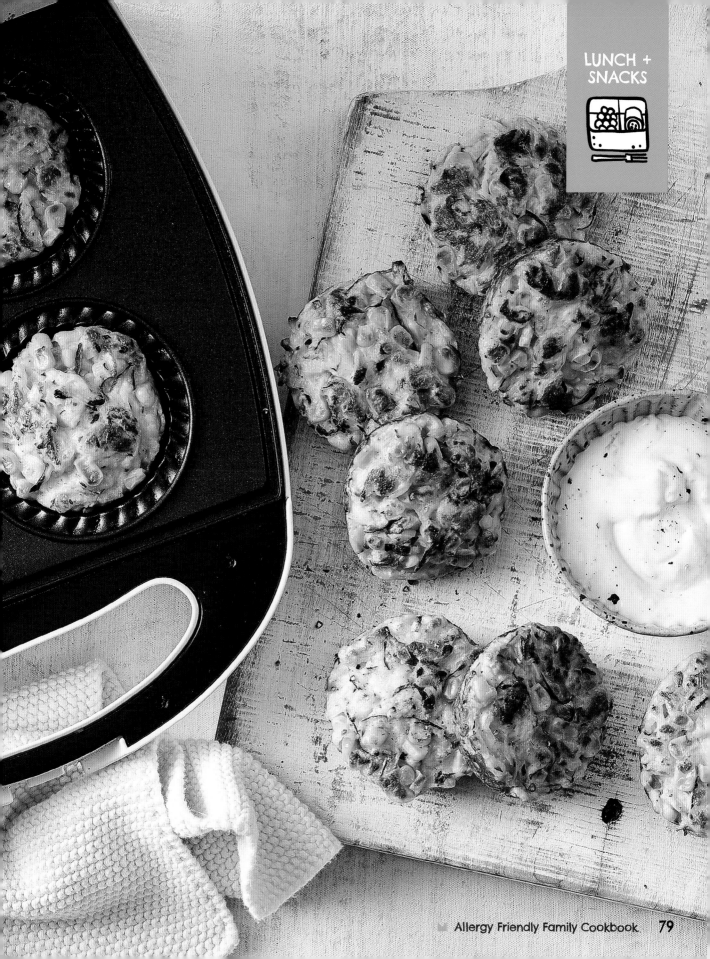

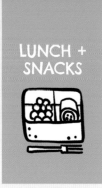

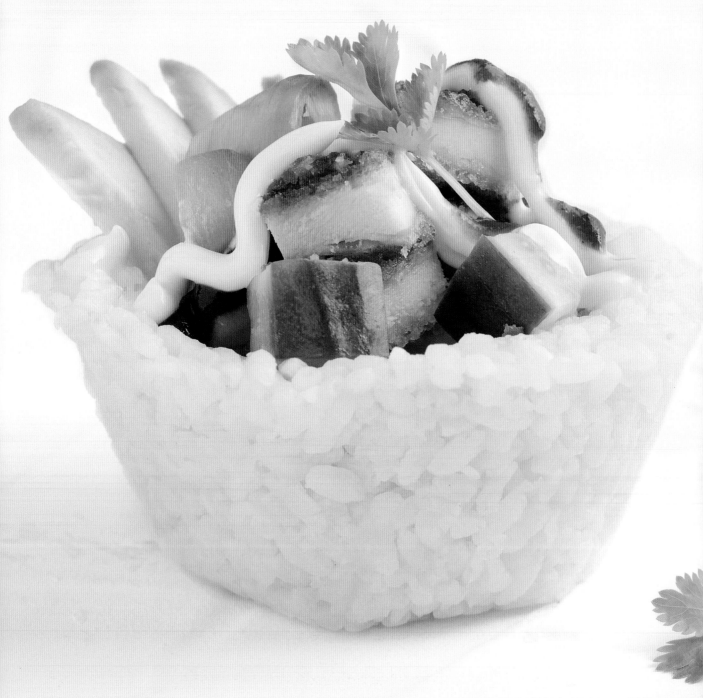

muffin pan
SUSHI CUPS

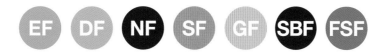

EF DF **NF** SF GF **SBF** FSF

It's super easy to perfect these cute sushi-inspired snacks. Just put your muffin pan to work and fill with your favourite bits and pieces.

makes 8   prep 10 mins (+ 15 mins chilling & 30 mins standing)   cook 15 mins

ingredients
215g (1 cup) sushi rice, rinsed well
60ml (¼ cup) sushi seasoning

1 Place the rice in a saucepan. Pour in 250ml (1 cup) water. Cover and set aside for 30 minutes to soak.

2 Meanwhile, cut eight 10cm-square pieces of baking paper. Use to line eight 80ml (⅓ cup) muffin pans. Bring rice to the boil over high heat. Cover, reduce heat to low and simmer for 15 minutes. Stand, covered, for 15 minutes to steam. Use a fork to fluff and separate the grains.

3 Evenly spread rice on a baking tray. Pour over sushi seasoning and use a spatula to fold through rice until mixture reaches room temperature.

4 Place 2 tbs rice in each prepared muffin pan. Press well into the base and up the side of each hole. Cool in the fridge for 15 minutes.

5 Transfer rice cups to a serving platter and gently remove the baking paper. Fill with your choice of filings (see below), to serve.

PER SERVE 2g protein, 0.3g fat (0g saturated fat), 22.7g carb, 0.3g dietary fibre, 103 Cals (432kJ)

make it your way FILL 'EM UP We used chopped chicken schnitzel, sliced cucumber and avocado, pickled ginger and a generous squirt of Kewpie mayo, but you can fill these cups with whatever suits your dietary needs.

smoked salmon
QUICHE CUPS

Gluten-free bread is the ideal pastry alternative in these mini salmon quiche cups, just perfect for a fancier light lunch or entertaining a crowd.

makes 12   prep 15 mins   cook 25 mins

ingredients

500g gluten-free sliced mixed seed loaf, crusts removed
2 tbs extra virgin olive oil
6 eggs
200g fresh ricotta, crumbled
80g (½ cup) frozen baby peas, thawed
¾ cup fresh dill sprigs, chopped
¼ cup finely chopped fresh chives
1 lemon, rind finely grated, juiced
2 small zucchini, peeled into ribbons
200g smoked salmon, torn

1 Preheat oven to 180°C/160°C fan forced. Grease twelve 80ml (⅓ cup) muffin pans with olive oil. Place the bread slices side-by-side on a flat surface. Use a rolling pin to flatten. Line the prepared pans with the bread slices. Brush with 1 tbs oil. Bake for 6 minutes or until light golden. Set aside to cool.

2 Combine the eggs, ricotta, peas, ½ cup dill, 2 tbs chives and lemon rind in a bowl. Season. Divide mixture among bread cups. Bake for 1 5 minutes or until just set. Cool slightly.

3 Place the zucchini, 1 tbs lemon juice and the remaining oil, dill and chives in a bowl. Season. Toss to combine. Add the salmon and gently toss to combine. Divide the zucchini mixture among the quiches and serve immediately.

PER SERVE 34g protein, 35g fat (8g saturated fat), 46g carb, 8g dietary fibre, 653 Cals (2734kJ)

make it your way
DAIRY FREE Swap the ricotta for vegan soy or coconut cheese.
FISH & SEAFOOD FREE Simply substitute the salmon for chopped ham or chorizo, or finely chopped barbecued chicken.

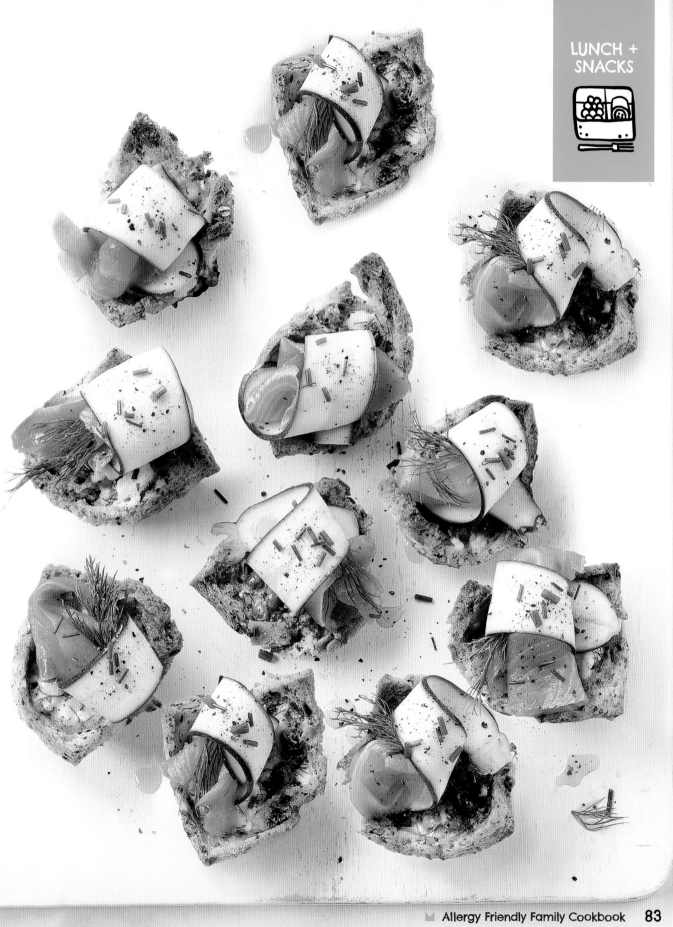

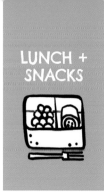

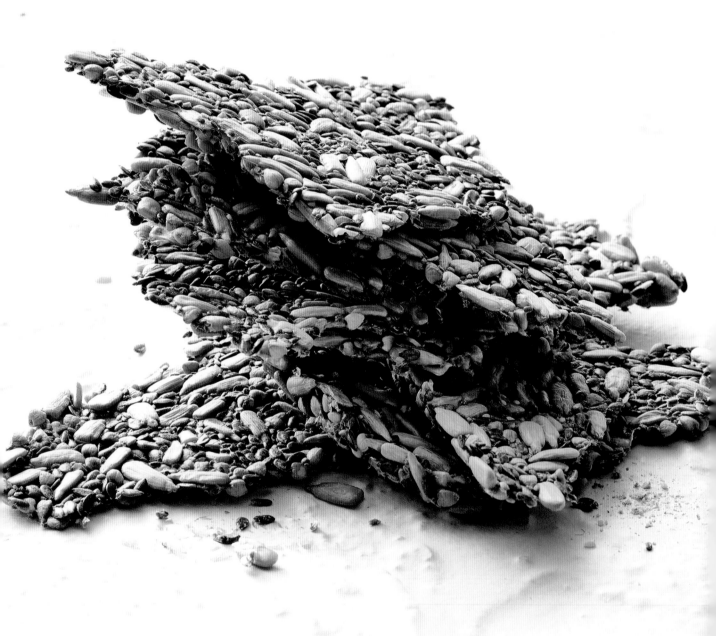

healthy seed CRACKERS

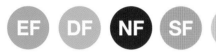

EF **DF** **NF** **SF** **GF** **SBF** **FSF**

Looking for a fast healthy snack to get you through the day? These crackers have seeds galore. They're just awaiting a tasty topping.

serves 6   prep 5 mins (+ cooling & 20 mins standing)   cook 1 hour

ingredients

230g (1½ cups) sunflower
  seed kernels
80g (½ cup) linseeds
110g (½ cup) raw buckwheat
40g (¼ cup) chia seeds
1 tsp salt
375ml (1½ cups) warm water

1 Preheat oven to 160°C/140°C fan forced. Line 2 baking trays with baking paper.

2 Combine all the ingredients in a large bowl. Set aside, stirring occasionally, for 20 minutes or until the water is absorbed.

3 Firmly press the seed mixture in a thin layer over each prepared tray, ensuring there are no gaps. Bake for 1 hour or until golden and crisp. Cool on trays. Break into large pieces. Store in an airtight container until ready to serve.

PER SERVE 14.3g protein, 27.8g fat (2.5g saturated fat), 12.2g carb, 11g dietary fibre, 375 Cals (1566kJ)

make it your way

TOP THEM These crackers taste amazing topped with avocado, tomato and vintage cheddar cheese, hummus, or smoked salmon and cream cheese. Use dairy-free cheeses, if needed.

mac 'n' cheese
ZUCCHINI SLICE

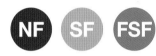

Two fan favourites — mac 'n' cheese and zucchini slice — combine in this tasty lunch-box filler or easy dinner idea. Enjoy it warmed up or not, it's up to you.

serves 6   prep 20 mins   cook 45 mins

ingredients

- 145g (1 cup) dried macaroni pasta
- 1 tbs extra virgin olive oil
- 1 small brown onion, finely chopped
- 2 garlic cloves, finely chopped
- 3 tsp fresh thyme leaves
- 125g middle bacon rashers, trimmed, chopped
- 2 zucchini, coarsely grated
- 200g orange sweet potato, unpeeled, coarsely grated
- 50g (⅓ cup) self-raising flour
- 4 eggs, lightly whisked
- 40g (½ cup) grated cheddar

1 Preheat oven to 180°C/160°C fan forced. Grease a 6cm-deep, 20cm (base size) square cake pan. Line base and sides with baking paper, extending paper 2cm above edges on all sides.

2 Cook pasta in salted boiling water following packet directions or until al dente. Drain. Refresh under cold water. Drain well.

3 Meanwhile, heat the oil in a frying pan over medium-high heat. Add the onion, garlic, thyme and bacon. Cook, stirring, for 5 minutes or until onion is softened. Add zucchini and sweet potato. Cook, stirring, for 5 minutes or until sweet potato is softened. Transfer to a large bowl.

4 Add the pasta, flour, eggs and half the cheese to the vegetable mixture. Season and stir to combine. Pour mixture into the prepared pan. Sprinkle with remaining cheese. Bake for 30-35 minutes or until golden and firm. Cool in the pan. Cut into squares, to serve.

PER SERVE 7.4g protein, 4.3g fat (1.3 saturated fat), 13.1g carb, 2g dietary fibre, 125 Cals (523kJ).

make it your way GLUTEN FREE Use gluten-free pasta and flour. SOY FREE Use soy-free flour. DAIRY FREE Use vegan cheese. BOOST Make a meal of it by serving with salad leaves, and chopped capsicum and carrot.

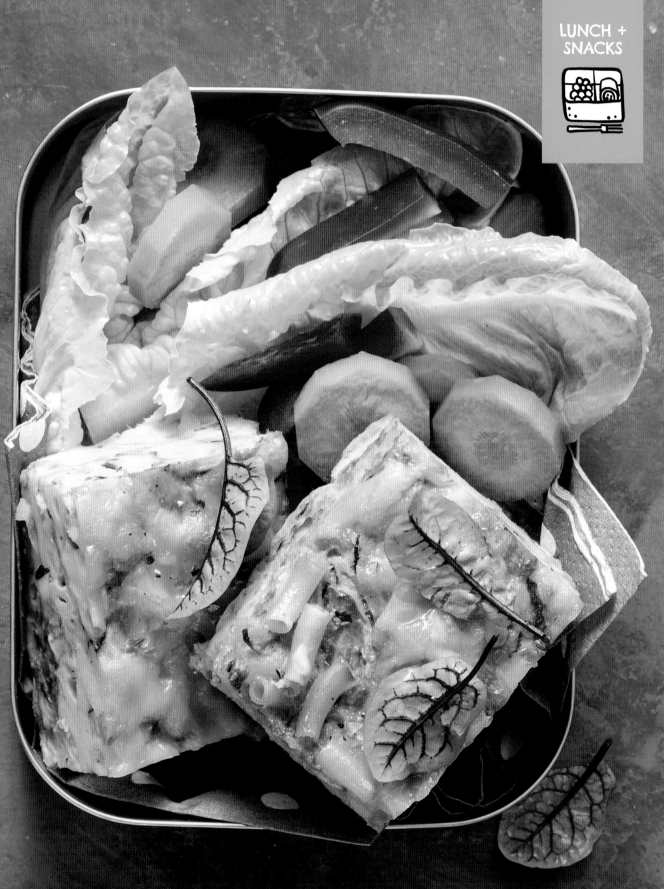

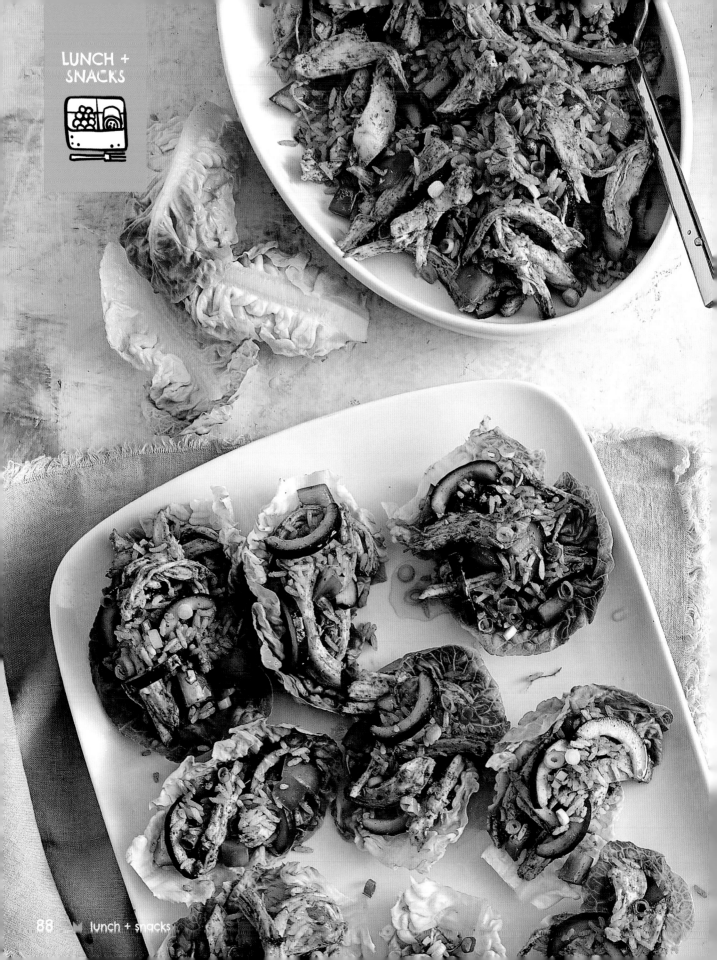

peri peri chicken
LETTUCE CUPS

These cute cups have just enough spice to entice — though you can tone that down for the young ones. Perfect for a light lunch or finger food.

serves 4   prep 15 mins   cook 5 mins

ingredients

25g sachet medium peri peri spice mix
200g (2 cups) shredded cooked chicken
250g pkt microwave 90-second long-grain white rice
1 Lebanese cucumber, halved lengthways, seeded, thinly sliced
1 green capsicum, finely chopped
2 green shallots, thinly sliced
2 tbs fresh lemon juice
1 tbs extra virgin olive oil
1 little gem lettuce, leaves separated

1 Combine the spice mix and chicken in a large microwave-safe bowl. Microwave for 1 minute or until warmed through.

2 Cook the rice following packet directions. Add rice to the chicken mixture with the cucumber, capsicum, shallot, lemon juice and oil. Toss until well combined. Divide among lettuce leaves, to serve.

PER SERVE 25.1g protein, 10.2g fat (1.6g saturated fat), 28.8g carb, 3.3g dietary fibre, 315 Cals (1318kJ)

make it your way

MAKE AHEAD Prepare the chicken mixture up to 2 days ahead of time. Store in an airtight container in the fridge. Simply top the lettuce cups with the mixture when you're ready to serve.

cheesy corn + capsicum
MUFFINS

Craving an afternoon snack? These savoury muffins will hit the spot.
The kids will love them as after-school hunger busters!

makes 12   prep 25 mins (+ cooling)   cook 30 mins

ingredients

500ml (2 cups) milk
170g (1 cup) instant polenta
2 tsp extra virgin olive oil
1 red capsicum, deseeded,
    finely chopped
300g can corn kernels, drained
2 green shallots, thinly sliced,
    plus extra, to serve
120g (1½ cups) cheddar,
    coarsely grated
130g (1 cup) gluten-free
    self-raising flour
2 tsp gluten-free baking powder
2 tsp gluten-free smoky BBQ
    seasoning
2 eggs, lightly whisked

1. Preheat oven to 200°C/180°C fan forced. Line twelve 80ml (⅓ cup) muffin pans with muffin cases.

2. Place 375ml (1½ cups) of milk in a small saucepan. Bring to a simmer over medium heat. Add the polenta and cook, stirring, for 1 minute. Set aside, stirring occasionally, until cooled slightly.

3. Meanwhile, heat the oil in a small frying pan over medium heat. Add capsicum. Cook, stirring occasionally, for 5 minutes or until softened. Transfer to a bowl. Toss in corn, shallot and cheese. Set aside.

4. Combine the flour, baking powder and seasoning in a large bowl. Make a well in the centre. Add egg, polenta mixture and remaining milk to the well. Season. Stir through half the capsicum mixture.

5. Divide mixture among prepared pans. Scatter with remaining capsicum mixture. Bake for 17 minutes or until golden and set. Cool. Sprinkle with extra shallot, to serve.

PER SERVE 7.1g protein, 6.8g fat (3.5g saturated fat), 24.9g carb, 1.4g dietary fibre, 193 Cals (805kJ)

make it your way

DAIRY FREE Use a plant-based nut- and soy-free milk, and opt for coconut cheese. EGG FREE Swap eggs for equivalent egg replacer.

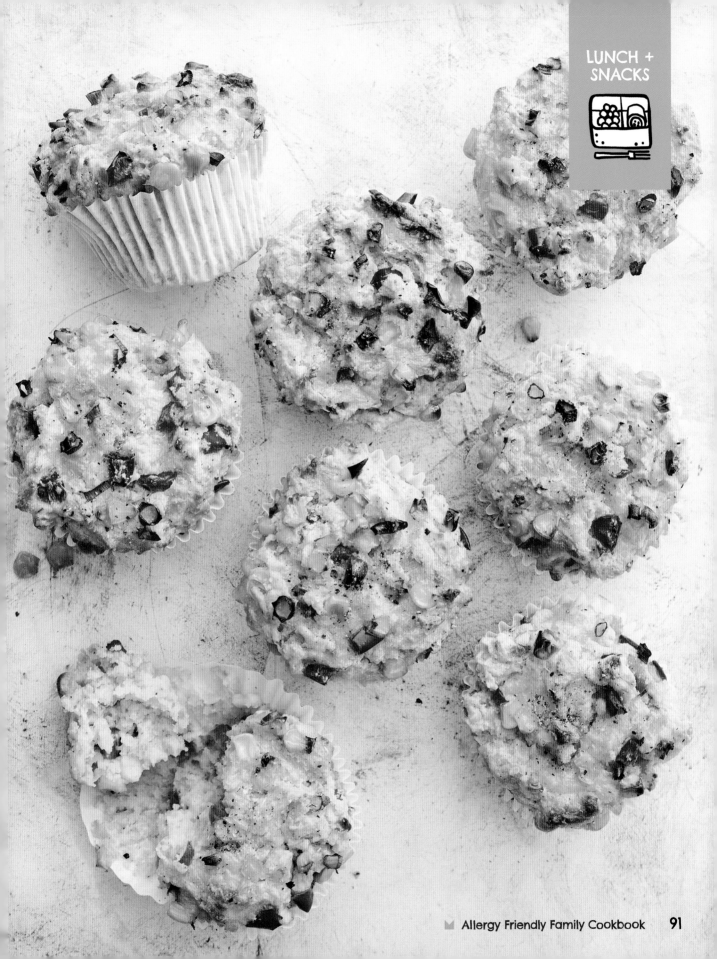

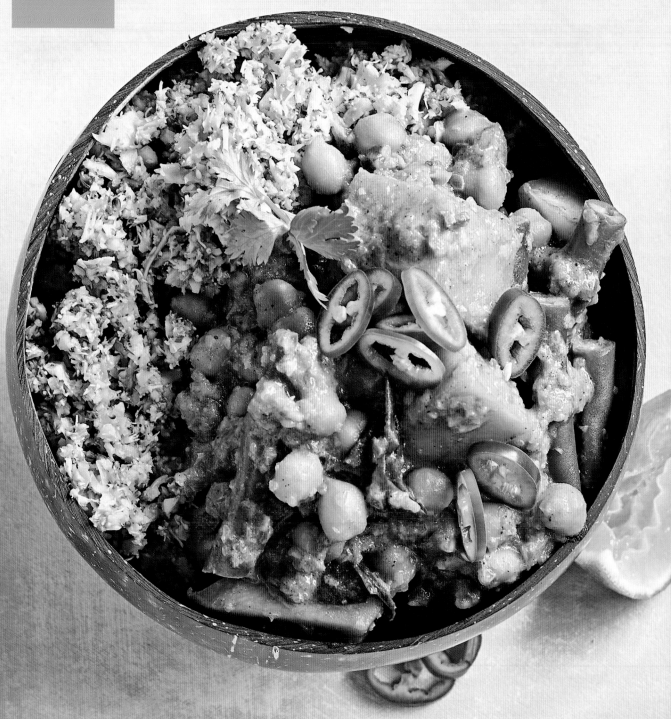

chickpea curry +
BROCCOLI RICE

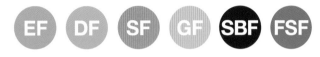

(EF) (DF) (SF) (GF) (SBF) (FSF)

This hearty low-calorie dish is packed with flavour and will warm you up on the chilliest of days. Start this recipe the day before serving.

serves 4   prep 20 mins (+ overnight soaking)   cook 1 hour 10 mins

ingredients

210g (1 cup) dried chickpeas
1 large red onion, chopped
3 garlic cloves, chopped
3cm-piece ginger, peeled, chopped
2 long fresh green chillies, chopped, plus extra chilli, sliced, to serve
1 tsp garam masala
2 tsp ground cumin
2 tsp macadamia oil
2 tomatoes, chopped
250ml (1 cup) salt-reduced vegetable stock
125ml (½ cup) light coconut milk
300g peeled pumpkin, chopped
200g green beans
1½ limes, cut into wedges
600g broccoli, chopped
Fresh coriander sprigs, to serve

1 Soak chickpeas in a large bowl of water overnight. Drain. Place in a large saucepan and cover with cold water. Bring to the boil. Reduce heat to low. Simmer for 30-40 minutes or until tender. Drain. Set aside.

2 Process the onion, garlic, ginger, chilli, garam masala and cumin in a small food processor until a thick paste forms. Heat the oil in a large saucepan or wok over medium heat. Add the paste. Cook, stirring, for 1-2 minutes or until aromatic. Add tomato and stir for 1 minute.

3 Add stock, coconut milk, chickpeas and pumpkin to the pan. Bring to the boil. Reduce heat to low. Cover and simmer for 20 minutes.

4 Meanwhile, cut beans into 4cm lengths. Add to the pan, cover and simmer for 5 minutes or until tender. Squeeze in 2 lime wedges.

5 Process the broccoli, in batches, in a food processor until coarse crumbs form. Steam or microwave until just tender. Drain and divide among serving bowls. Top with curry, coriander and extra chilli. Serve with the remaining lime wedges.

PER SERVE 25g protein, 7g fat (3g saturated fat), 38g carb, 19g dietary fibre, 363 Cals (1517kJ)

make it your way

NUT FREE Swap macadamia oil for extra virgin olive oil or vegetable oil.
TRY Add chopped barbecued chicken to pan in Step 4. Heat through.

sweet potato + thyme
WRAPS

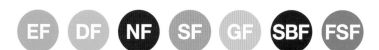

With only five ingredients, these wraps are just so easy to make, and you won't even notice they are gluten free. Fill them up however you like.

makes 8   prep 20 mins (+ 10 mins cooling)   cook 30 mins

ingredients

150g orange sweet potato, peeled, grated
375g (2½ cups) gluten-free and soy-free white bread mix
1 tsp salt
1 tbs coarsely chopped fresh thyme leaves
1 tbs extra virgin olive oil

1 Place the sweet potato in a microwave-safe bowl. Cover and microwave for 3-4 minutes or until just tender. Cool for 10 minutes.

2 Combine the bread mix, salt, thyme and cooled sweet potato in a large bowl. Season with pepper. Add 410ml (1⅔ cups) water. Whisk until smooth and combined. (The batter may thicken upon standing; add a little water, if needed.)

3 Brush a large frying pan with a little oil and heat over medium heat. Spoon ⅓ cup batter into the pan. Use a palette knife to spread batter into a 20cm round. Cook for 2 minutes or until golden underneath. Turn over. Cook for 1 minute or until cooked through and golden underneath. Wrap in a clean tea towel to cool. Repeat with the remaining batter to make 8 wraps. Store wraps in a sealable bag in the fridge for up to 3 days.

PER SERVE 29.7g protein, 8.9g fat (2.3g saturated fat), 29.1g carb, 11.4g dietary fibre, 343 Cals (1432kJ)

make it your way
FILL 'EM Try torn cos lettuce leaves, sliced tomato, Lebanese cucumber and pitted kalamata olives, fresh continental parsley leaves, drained and flaked tuna in oil, and gluten- and dairy-free tzatziki.

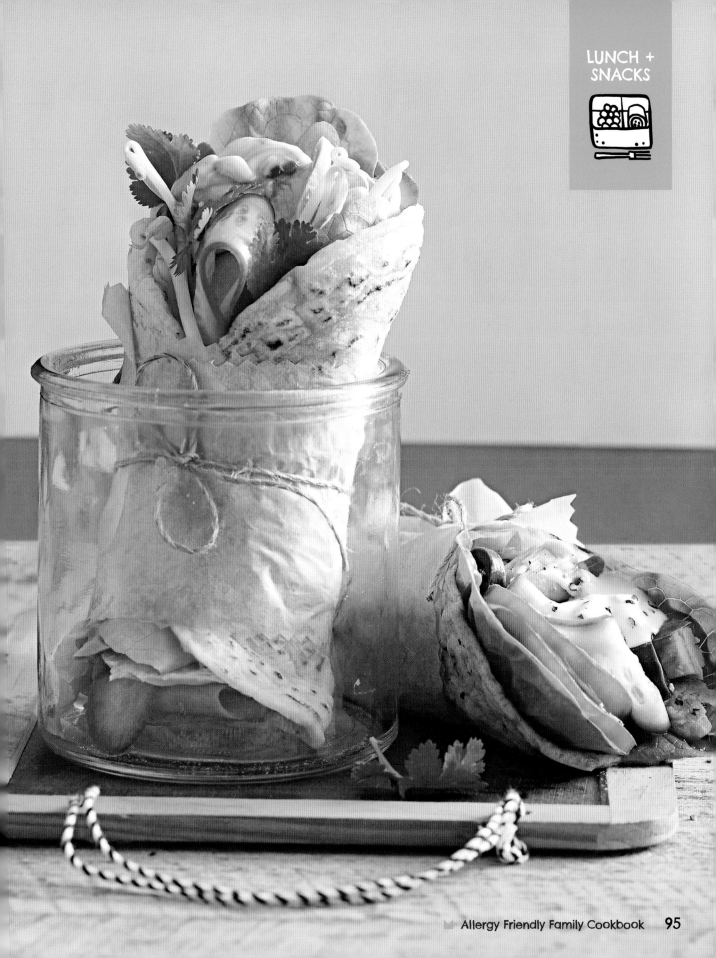

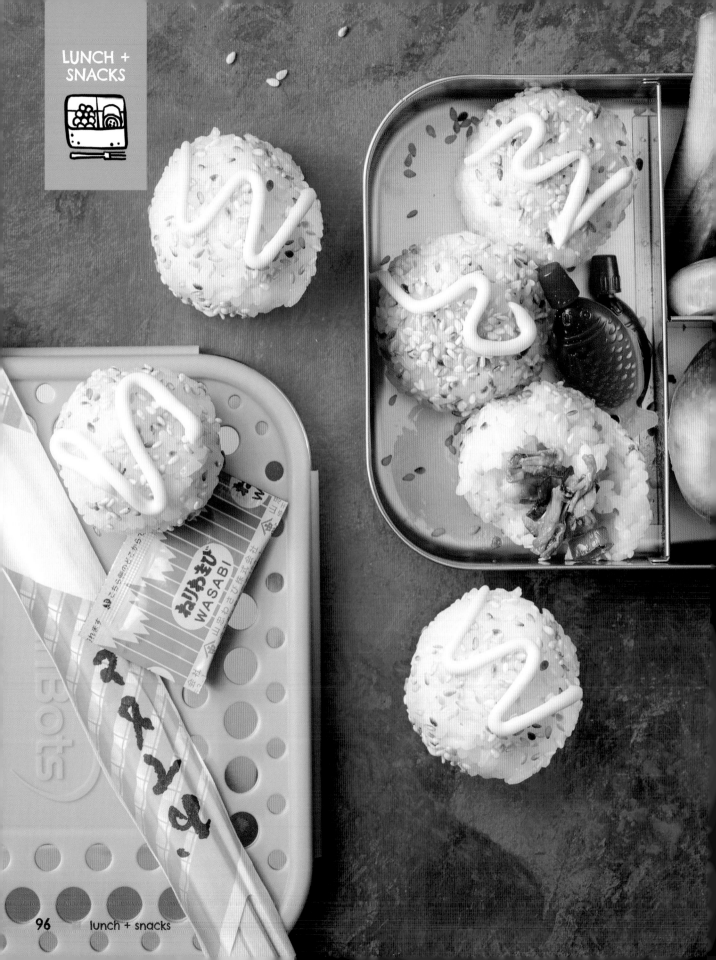

teriyaki sushi chicken
RICE BALLS

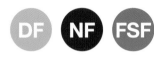

These teriyaki chicken balls are quick and easy to prepare.
The kids will adore them in their lunch boxes or as a filling snack.

makes 22   prep 40 mins (+ 10 mins standing & 10 mins cooling)   cook 25 mins

ingredients

430g (2 cups) sushi rice, rinsed
   and drained
80ml (⅓ cup) rice wine vinegar
1 tbs caster sugar
1 tsp salt
2 tsp vegetable oil
250g chicken tenderloins
60ml (¼ cup) teriyaki sauce
1 green shallot, thinly sliced
2 tbs sesame seeds, toasted
Kewpie mayonnaise, wasabi
   and salt-reduced soy sauce,
   to serve

1   Place rice in a saucepan with 500ml (2 cups) water. Bring to the boil over high heat. Reduce heat to low. Cover. Simmer for 15 minutes or until water absorbs. Remove from heat. Stand, covered, for 10 minutes.

2   Transfer rice to a large glass or ceramic bowl. Gently fold in vinegar, sugar and salt until cooled. Cover with a damp tea towel. Set aside.

3   Meanwhile, heat the oil in a small non-stick frying pan over medium-high heat. Add chicken. Cook, turning, for 5 minutes or until almost cooked through. Add sauce. Cook, turning chicken, for 2-3 minutes or until chicken is cooked through and sauce thickens. Transfer chicken to a board and finely chop. Place in a small bowl with the shallot and any pan juices. Stir to combine. Cool for 10 minutes.

4   Using damp hands and 1 rounded tbs rice at a time, firmly shape rice into 22 balls. One at a time, press a finger into a ball to form a hole. Fill with a little chicken mixture, then shape surrounding rice to cover mixture. Place on a plate. Sprinkle with sesame seeds. Place in fridge until required. Serve with mayonnaise, wasabi and soy sauce.

PER BALL 4.2g protein, 2.7g fat (0.4g saturated fat), 16.9g carb, 0.5g dietary fibre, 111 Cals (464kJ)   .

make it your way   EGG FREE Use egg-free or vegan mayo, to serve. SESAME FREE Omit the sesame seeds and roll the balls in nigella seeds, if you like.

tuna, corn + chive
TARTLETS

Good things come in small packages, and these gluten-free mini tartlets are the perfect example. So many delicious flavours in one bite.

makes 24   prep 20 mins (+ standing)   cook 20 mins

ingredients

Rice flour, to dust

3 sheets savoury gluten-free shortcrust pastry, just thawed

185g can tuna in springwater, drained, flaked

100g (½ cup) frozen corn kernels, thawed

2 tbs finely chopped fresh chives

½ red capsicum, finely chopped

30g grated reduced-fat cheddar

3 eggs

125ml (½ cup) milk

1 Preheat oven to 190°C/170°C fan forced. Lightly grease two 12-hole, 60ml (1½ tbs) round-based patty pans. Dust holes with rice flour, shaking out excess.

2 Use a 7.5cm round cutter to cut 24 rounds from the pastry sheets. Press each round firmly into the prepared holes.

3 Place the tuna, corn, chives, capsicum and cheese in a bowl. Whisk eggs and milk in a jug. Add to the tuna mixture. Season and stir to combine. Spoon 1 tbs filling into each pastry case. Bake for 15-20 minutes or until golden and puffed. Stand for 5 minutes. Serve.

PER TARTLET 4g protein, 6.8g fat (3g saturated fat), 11.9g carb, 0.5g dietary fibre, 126 Cals (529kJ)

make it your way DAIRY FREE Simply use a plant-based milk instead of cow's milk, and vegan cheese in place of the cheddar. TRY THIS Instead of the tuna, use 185g chopped gluten-free premium ham.

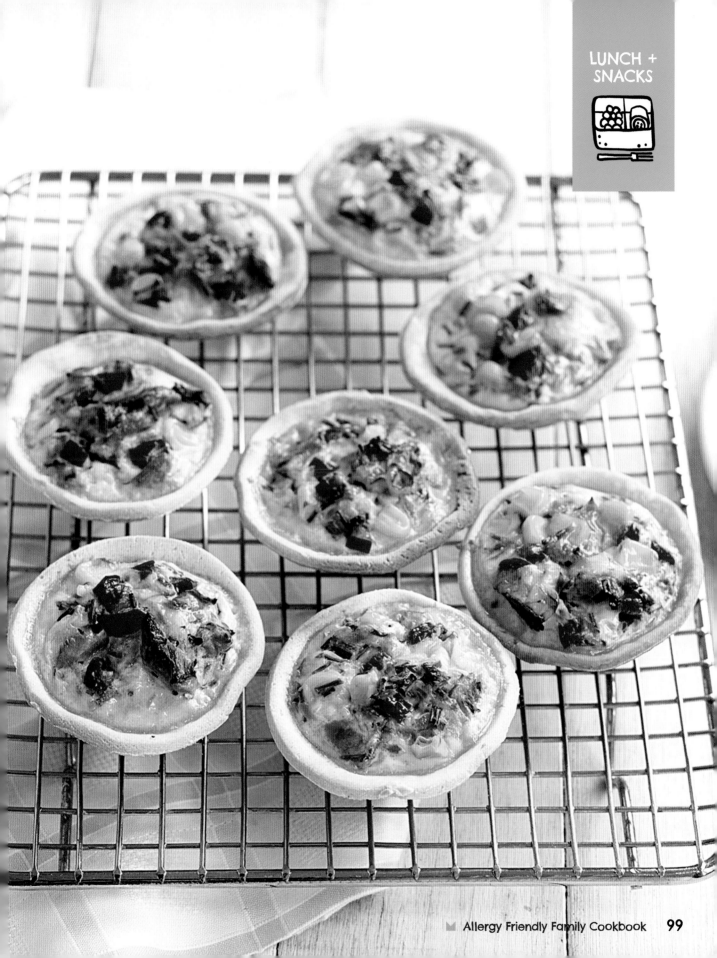

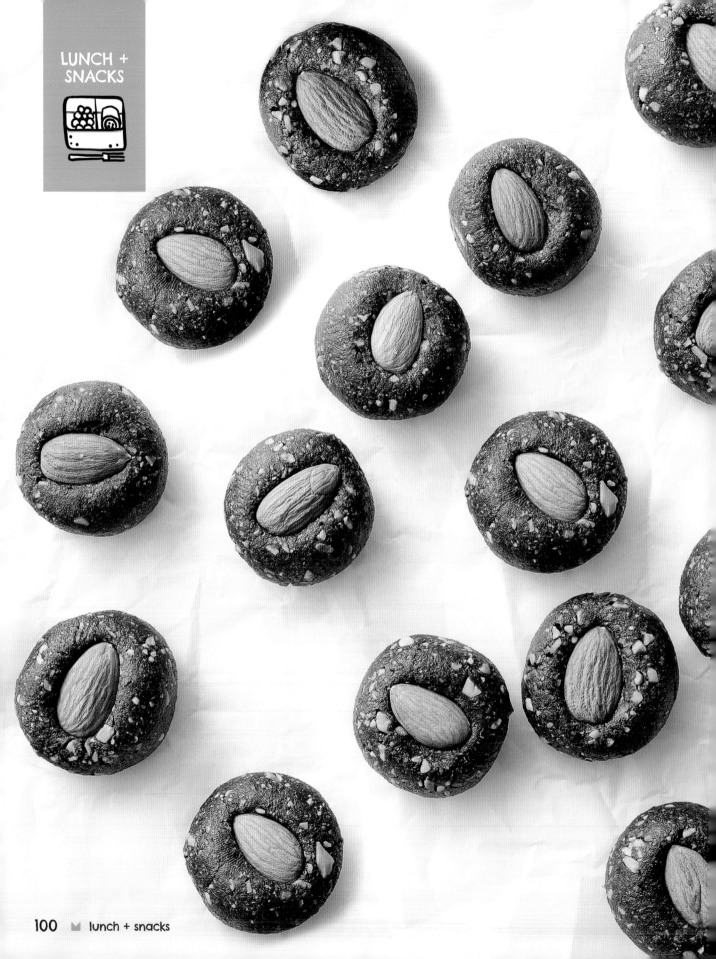

no-bake
RAWIES

These easy no-bake treats are a fun, better-for-you way to snack. They keep for a while, so why not make a double batch?

makes 30   prep 10 mins

ingredients

400g pitted medjool dates
85g (1 cup) desiccated coconut
35g (⅓ cup) cocoa powder
90g (⅔ cup) dry-roasted
   almonds, plus an extra 30,
   to decorate
1 tsp ground cinnamon
2 tsp vanilla extract

1 Place the dates, coconut, cocoa, almonds, cinnamon and vanilla in a food processor and process until well combined.

2 Roll level tablespoonfuls of mixture into balls and place on a tray. Flatten each ball slightly. Press a roasted almond in the centre of each flattened ball. Serve.

PER SERVE 1.5g protein, 3.1g fat (1.1g saturated fat), 13.7g carb, 2.1g dietary fibre, 82 Cals (343kJ)

make it your way
SAVE FOR LATER Place the rawies in an airtight container in the fridge for up to 2 weeks. TRY THIS Instead of using almonds, add roasted pecans or peanuts.

simply free apricot
BLISS BALLS

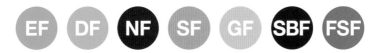

(EF) (DF) (**NF**) (SF) (GF) (**SBF**) (FSF)

Send the kids to school with these healthier bliss balls packed with dates, carrots, oats and dried apricot. And don't forget to save some for yourself, too!

makes 25   prep 25 mins (+ 15 mins soaking)

ingredients
200g dried apricots,
   coarsely chopped
2 tbs white chia seeds
125ml (½ cup) fresh orange juice
10 medjool dates, pitted
75g (¾ cup) gluten-free
   rolled oats
70g (½ cup) grated carrot
2 tbs moist coconut flakes,
   plus an extra 20g (⅓ cup)
Pinch of ground cinnamon

1 Combine the apricot, chia and orange juice in a shallow dish. Set aside, stirring occasionally, for 15 minutes to soak.

2 Transfer the apricot mixture to a food processor. Add the dates, oats, carrot, coconut and cinnamon. Process until finely chopped and evenly combined.

3 Place the extra coconut on a plate. Roll level tablespoonfuls of the mixture into balls and roll in the coconut. Serve.

PER BALL 1.2g protein, 1.1g fat (0.5g saturated fat), 13.2g carb, 2.3g dietary fibre, 69 Cals (288kJ)

make it your way MAKE AHEAD Keep the balls in an airtight container in the fridge for up to 4 days. FREEZE IT Batch-freeze the balls in airtight containers for up to 1 month. Thaw in the fridge before eating.

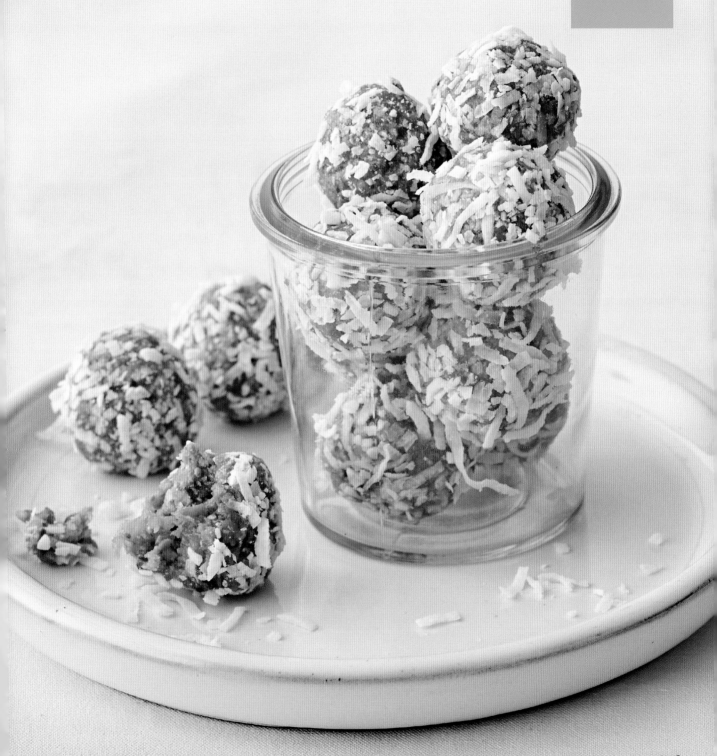

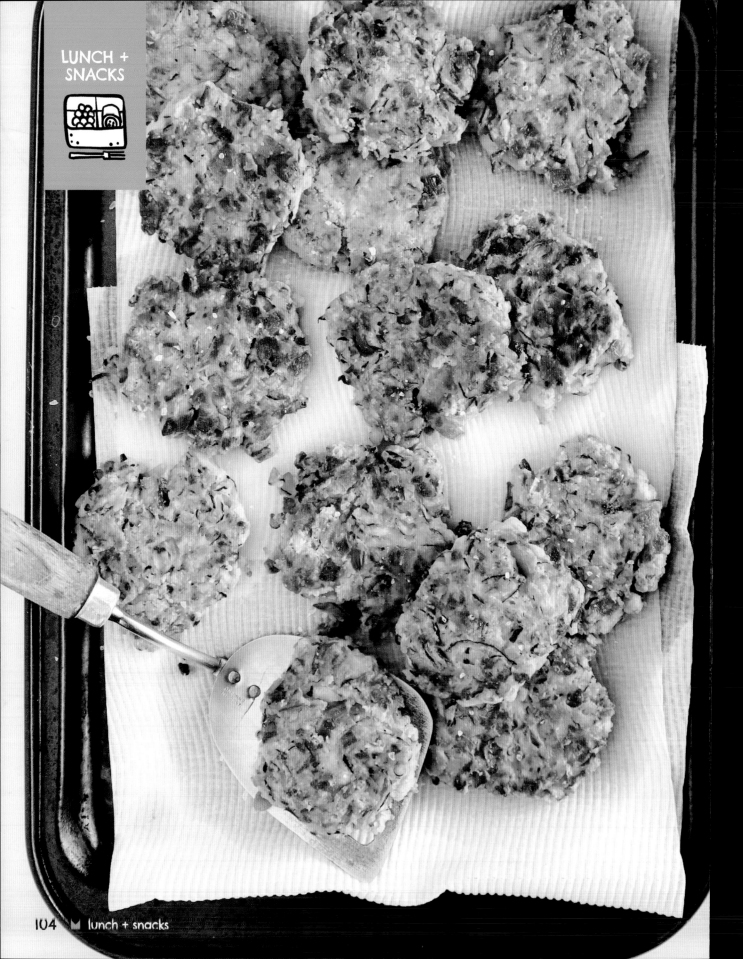

community recipe
zucchini
FRITTERS

 EF DF NF SF SBF FSF

"These are just like cook Lidia Bastianich's frittelle di zucchini. They are delicious hot or cold, and the nutritional yeast adds extra flavour. Take care when handling and turning. As they are not bound with egg, they can be a bit fragile and crumbly." ~ *Frances Oppedisano*

makes 18   **prep** 20 mins (+ standing & cooling)   **cook** 25 mins

ingredients

500g (about 2 large) zucchini, coarsely grated
1 tsp salt
2 tsp garlic olive oil
1 small red onion, finely chopped
150g (1 cup) plain flour
1½ tsp baking powder
20g (¼ cup) nutritional yeast flakes
60g (¼ cup) dairy-free margarine, melted
Canola or rice bran oil, to cook

1 Place zucchini in a large bowl. Add salt and toss to combine. Stand for 10 minutes. Use hands to squeeze excess liquid from the zucchini and return to the bowl.

2 Meanwhile, heat the garlic oil in a large non-stick frying pan over medium heat. Add the onion and cook, stirring occasionally, for 5 minutes or until softened. Cool.

3 Add the onion, flour, baking powder, yeast and margarine to the bowl. Stir to combine. Fill the frying pan with oil to about 3mm and heat over medium heat. Working in 2-3 batches, drop heaped tbs of mixture into the pan and press gently to flatten. Cook for 2 minutes each side or until golden. Drain on paper towel. Serve.

PER SERVE 5.3g protein, 18g fat (2.8g saturated fat), 21.9g carb, 2.7g dietary fibre, 274 Cals (1145kJ)

 make it your way   **GLUTEN FREE** Replace the plain flour with gluten-free plain flour.
BOOST Serve fritters with sweet chilli sauce for dipping.

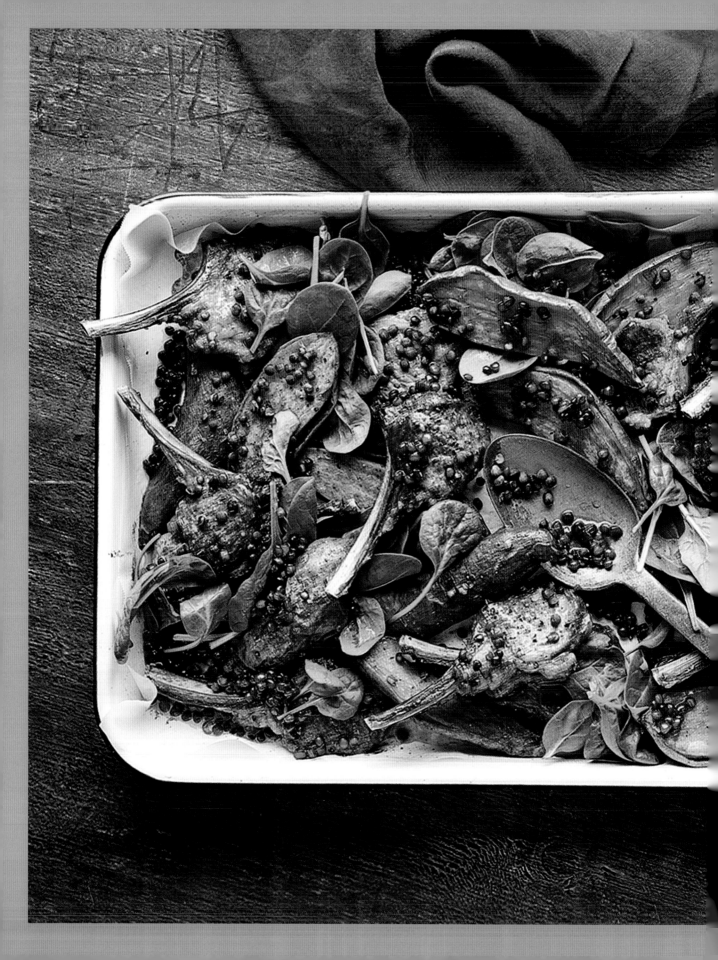

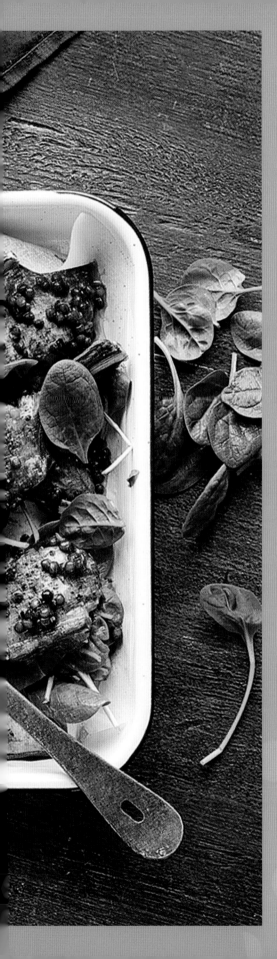

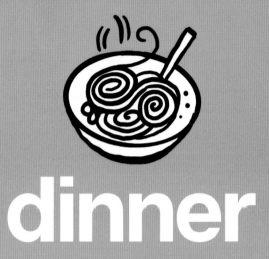

dinner

We've got you covered every night of week for when they ask: "What's for dinner?"

slow-cooker honey soy
DRUMSTICKS

Slow cooking these sticky chicken drumsticks makes them tender and fall off the bone, not to mention finger-lickin' good for a fun family dinner!

serves 4   prep 15 mins   cook 3 hours 5 mins

ingredients

125ml (½ cup) salt-reduced tamari sauce
80g (⅓ cup) honey
80ml (⅓ cup) gluten-free chicken stock
2cm-piece fresh ginger, finely grated
2 garlic cloves, crushed
2 tsp sesame oil
8 chicken drumsticks
2 tsp sesame seeds, toasted
Steamed long-grain white rice, Asian greens, thinly sliced green shallot and sliced red chilli, to serve

1 Combine the tamari sauce, honey, stock, ginger, garlic and oil in a slow cooker. Season with pepper.

2 Place the chicken in the slow cooker and toss to coat in the sauce mixture. Cover. Cook on High for 3 hours (or Low for 6 hours), turning drumsticks halfway through cooking, or until chicken is tender and cooked through.

3 Preheat an oven grill on high. Line a large baking tray with foil. Transfer chicken to prepared tray. Drizzle with a little of the cooking sauce. Grill, basting with extra sauce halfway through, for 2-3 minutes or until just starting to char.

4 Sprinkle chicken with sesame seeds. Serve with rice, Asian greens, shallot, chilli and the remaining cooking sauce.

PER SERVE 49.9g protein, 25.3g fat (7g saturated fat), 86.9g carb, 4.3g dietary fibre, 783 Cals (3275kJ)

make it your way
SOY FREE Swap the tamari sauce for coconut aminos sauce.
SESAME FREE Omit the sesame seeds and replace the sesame oil with avocado or perilla oil.

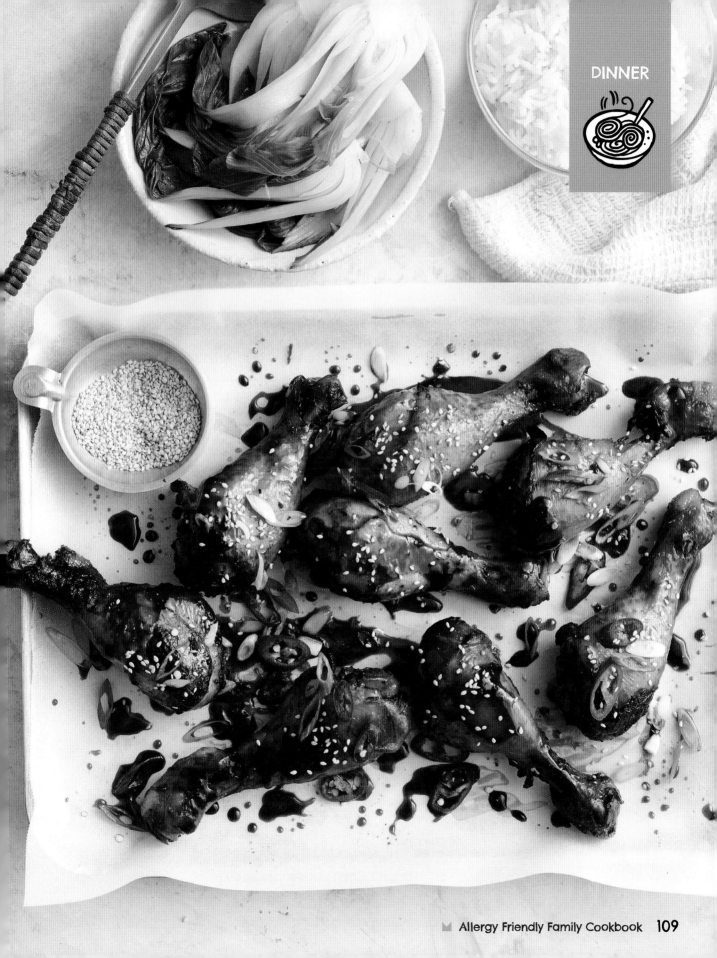

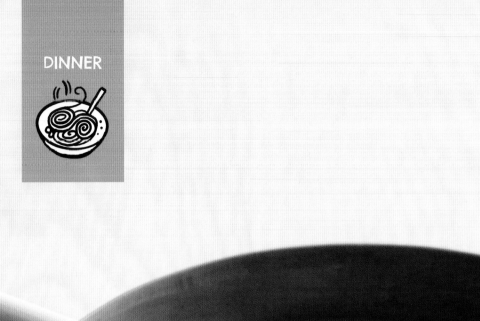

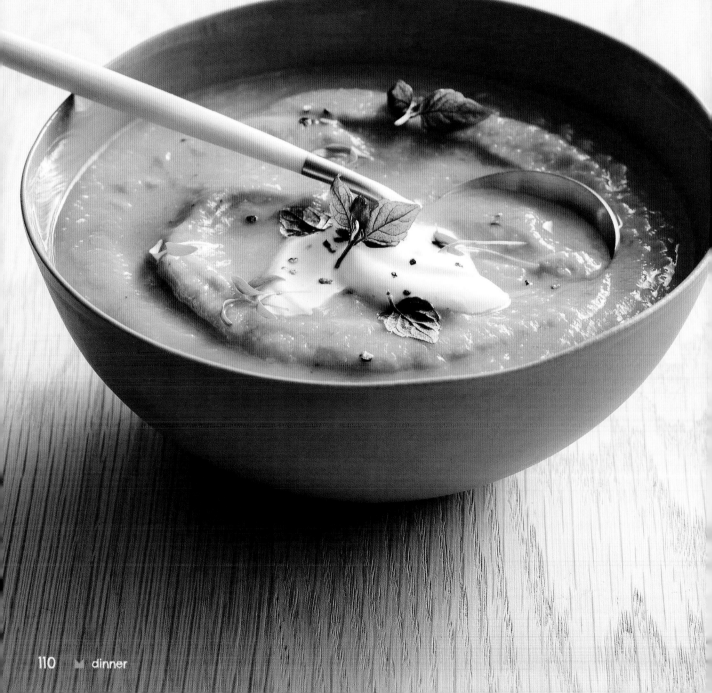

spicy roasted
PUMPKIN SOUP

Spiced up with ginger and turmeric, you'll definitely want a second bowl of this easy and delicious pumpkin soup.

serves 4   prep 25 mins (+ cooling)   cook 1 hour 35 mins

ingredients

1.6kg butternut pumpkin or
   kent pumpkin
60ml (¼ cup) olive oil
1 large brown onion,
   finely chopped
1-2 garlic cloves, finely chopped
1L (4 cups) gluten-free
   chicken stock
1 tbs finely grated fresh ginger
1 tbs finely grated fresh turmeric
Natural yoghurt and mixed
   baby herbs (such as
   coriander, purple radish
   sprouts), to serve

1. Preheat oven to 200°C/180°C fan forced. Line 2 baking trays with baking paper. Coarsely chop the pumpkin, including the seeds and skin, and spread on the prepared trays. Drizzle with 2 tbs oil. Bake for 1 hour 10 minutes or until pumpkin is soft and lightly coloured.

2. Heat the remaining oil in a large, heavy-based saucepan over medium heat. Add the onion. Cook, stirring, for 3-5 minutes or until softened. Add the garlic and cook, stirring, for 1 minute or until aromatic.

3. Add cooked pumpkin and juices from the tray to the pan. Pour in the stock. Bring to a simmer over medium-low heat. Simmer for 15 minutes. Stir in the ginger and turmeric. Remove from the heat. Cool slightly. Use a stick blender to puree the soup until smooth, thinning with a little water, if you prefer. Ladle soup among serving bowls. Dollop with yoghurt and sprinkle with herbs, to serve.

PER SERVE 16g protein, 19g fat (9g saturated fat), 31g carb,
9g dietary fibre, 373 Cals (1561kJ)

make it your way

DAIRY FREE Substitute the natural yoghurt for vegan coconut yoghurt. BOOST Add 2 halved carrots to the tray in step 1.

fabulous
FISH PIE

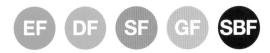

The winning combination of crispy and creamy make this gluten- and dairy-free fish pie a firm favourite.

serves 4   prep 30 mins   cook 55 mins

ingredients

400g cauliflower, cut into
   small florets
20g (¼ cup) nutritional
   yeast flakes
2 tsp cornflour
250ml (1 cup) unsweetened
   almond milk
60ml (¼ cup) extra virgin olive oil
1 leek, trimmed, sliced
1 carrot, peeled, chopped
2 celery stalks, chopped
800g red potatoes, peeled
500g skinless ling fish fillets
200g skinless salmon fillet
10 cooked small king prawns,
   peeled, deveined
1 tbs drained baby capers, rinsed
50g baby spinach
2 tbs coarsely chopped fresh
   dill, plus extra, to serve

1. Place cauliflower in a microwave-safe bowl. Add 1 tbs water. Cover. Microwave for 5-6 minutes or until very tender. Drain. Transfer to a food processor. Add yeast, cornflour and milk. Process until smooth.

2. Meanwhile, heat 2 tbs oil in a frying pan over medium-low heat. Add the leek. Cook, stirring occasionally, for 5 minutes or until softened. Add carrot and celery. Cook, stirring occasionally, for 10 minutes or until tender. Remove from the heat. Stir in the cauliflower mixture.

3. Grate potato into a sieve. Use the back of a large spoon to squeeze out excess moisture. Transfer to a bowl. Stir in remaining oil.

4. Preheat oven to 200°C/180°C fan forced. Grease a deep, 20 x 26cm (base size) baking dish. Cut ling into 4cm pieces and salmon into 3cm pieces. Add to prepared dish with the prawns, capers, spinach and dill. Pour over vegie mixture. Season well. Stir to combine. Evenly top with potato mixture. Season. Bake for 30-35 minutes or until golden and the seafood is cooked. Serve sprinkled with extra dill.

PER SERVE 61.5g protein, 23.8g fat (4.1g saturated fat), 30.9g carb, 10.5g dietary fibre, 617 Cals (2583kJ)

make it your way

NUT FREE Replace the almond milk with a nut-free milk, such as soy milk (contains soy) or cow's milk (contains dairy).

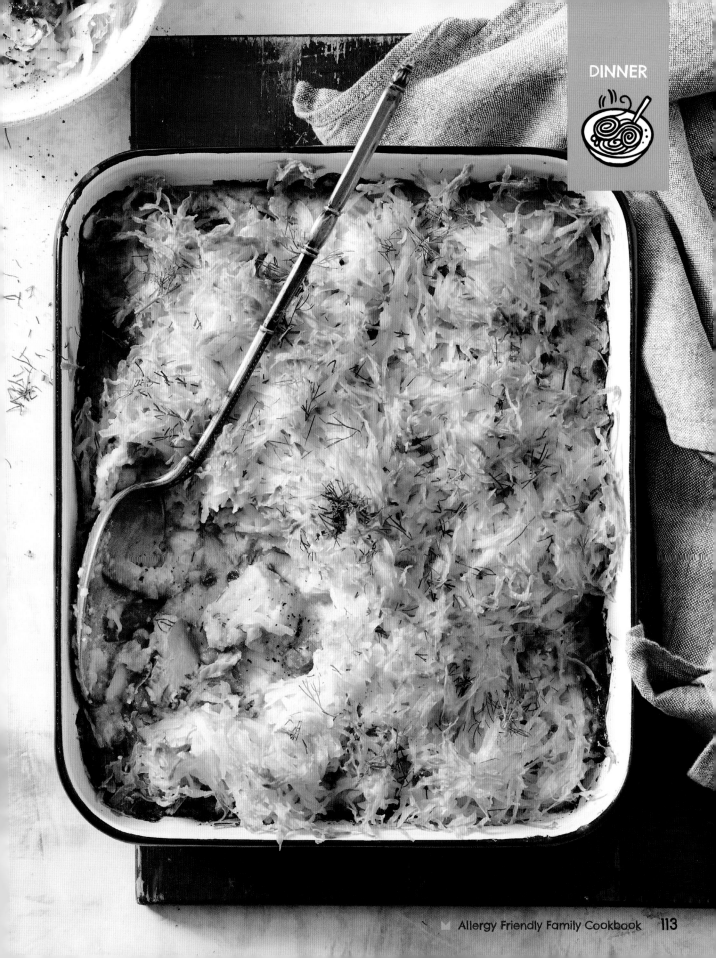

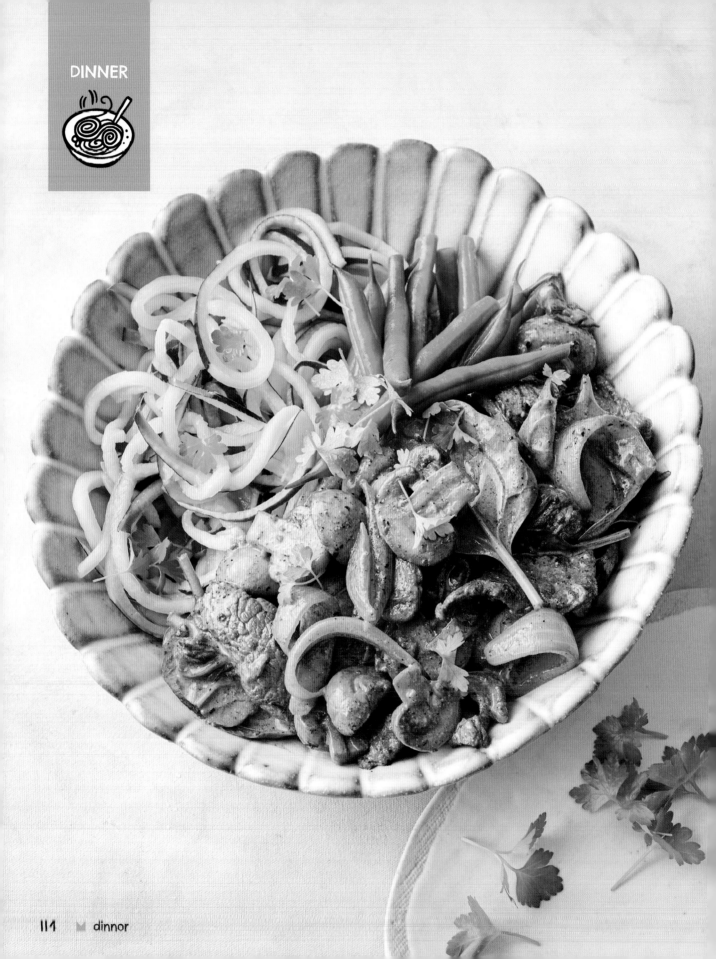

DINNER

better-for-you beef
STROGANOFF

We've given the classic beef stroganoff a healthy makeover using vegie noodles, light sour cream and salt-reduced stock, and it tastes great!

serves 4   prep 20 mins   cook 25 mins

ingredients

2 tsp olive oil

500g beef fillet, fat trimmed, thinly sliced

1 white onion, thinly sliced

200g Swiss brown mushrooms, halved or sliced

200g button mushrooms, halved or sliced

2 garlic cloves, crushed

1 tsp paprika

1 tbs gluten- and soy-free Worcestershire sauce

200ml salt-reduced gluten-free beef stock

60ml (¼ cup) light sour cream

100g baby spinach

2 x 250g pkt zucchini noodles

Steamed green beans and fresh continental parsley leaves, to serve

1 Heat 1 tsp oil in a large frying pan over high heat. In 2 batches, add beef and cook, stirring, for 2 minutes or until golden. Transfer to a plate.

2 Heat the remaining oil in the pan over medium heat. Add the onion and cook, stirring, for 5 minutes or until softened. Add mushrooms and increase heat to high. Cook, stirring, for 3-4 minutes or until browned. Add garlic and paprika. Cook, stirring, for 1 minute or until aromatic. Stir in Worcestershire sauce and stock. Bring to the boil.

3 Reduce heat to low, return beef to the pan and gently simmer for 1-2 minutes or until heated through. Stir through the sour cream and spinach, and cook until spinach has just wilted.

4 Microwave zucchini noodles following packet directions. Divide beef, zucchini noodles and steamed green beans among serving bowls. Sprinkled with parsley, to serve.

PER SERVE 35g protein, 13g fat (5g saturated fat), 6g carb, 5g dietary fibre, 297 Cals (1243kJ)

 make it your way

DAIRY FREE Use dairy-free sour cream. BOOST Serve stroganoff with cooked fettuccine or long-grain rice instead of zucchini noodles.

maple-glazed lamb
TRAY BAKE

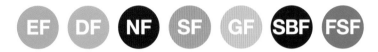

Sunday roasts aren't just for weekends. With only five ingredients, and by using lamb cutlets, this roast lamb cooks quick enough to enjoy during the week.

serves 4   prep 5 mins   cook 40 mins

ingredients

500g small sweet potatoes, scrubbed, quartered lengthways
12 French-trimmed lamb cutlets
400g can brown lentils, rinsed, drained
60ml (¼ cup) maple syrup
100g baby spinach

1 Preheat oven to 200°C/180°C fan forced. Line a large shallow baking tray with baking paper. Arrange sweet potato on the prepared tray. Spray with olive oil. Season. Bake for 20 minutes or until just tender.

2 Add the lamb and lentils to the tray. Spray with a little more oil and drizzle with maple syrup. Bake for 15-20 minutes or until the sweet potato is golden and the lamb is cooked to your liking. Stir through the spinach, to serve.

PER SERVE 28g protein, 11g fat (3g saturated fat), 22g carb, 5g dietary fibre, 447 Cals (1869kJ)

make it your way

SWAP IT You could replace the brown lentils for canned chickpeas, and the sweet potato for pumpkin, if you like.

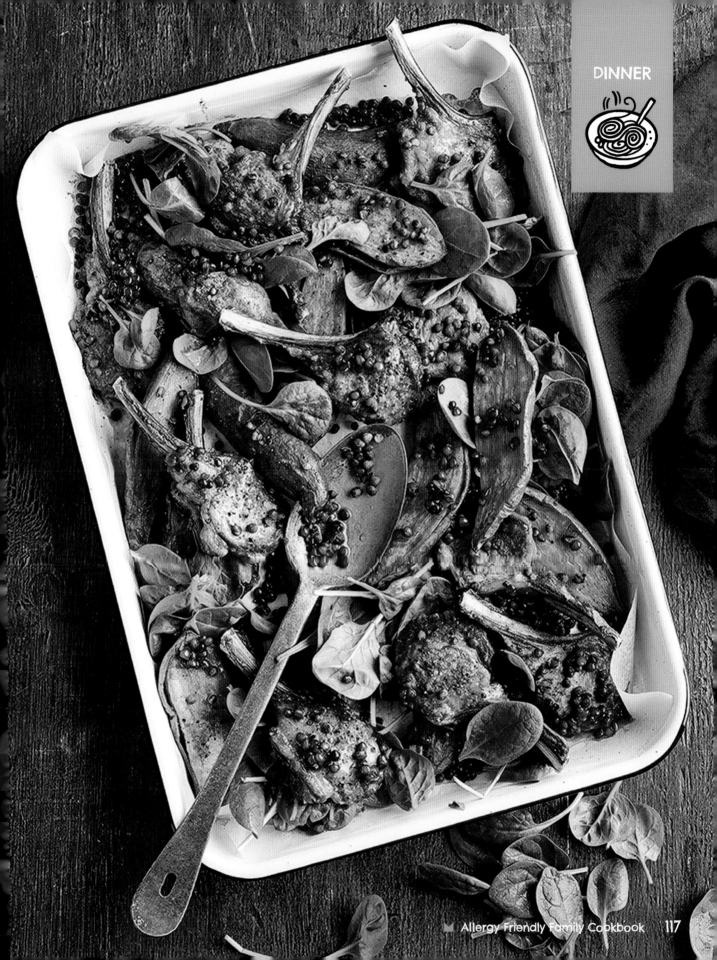

DINNER

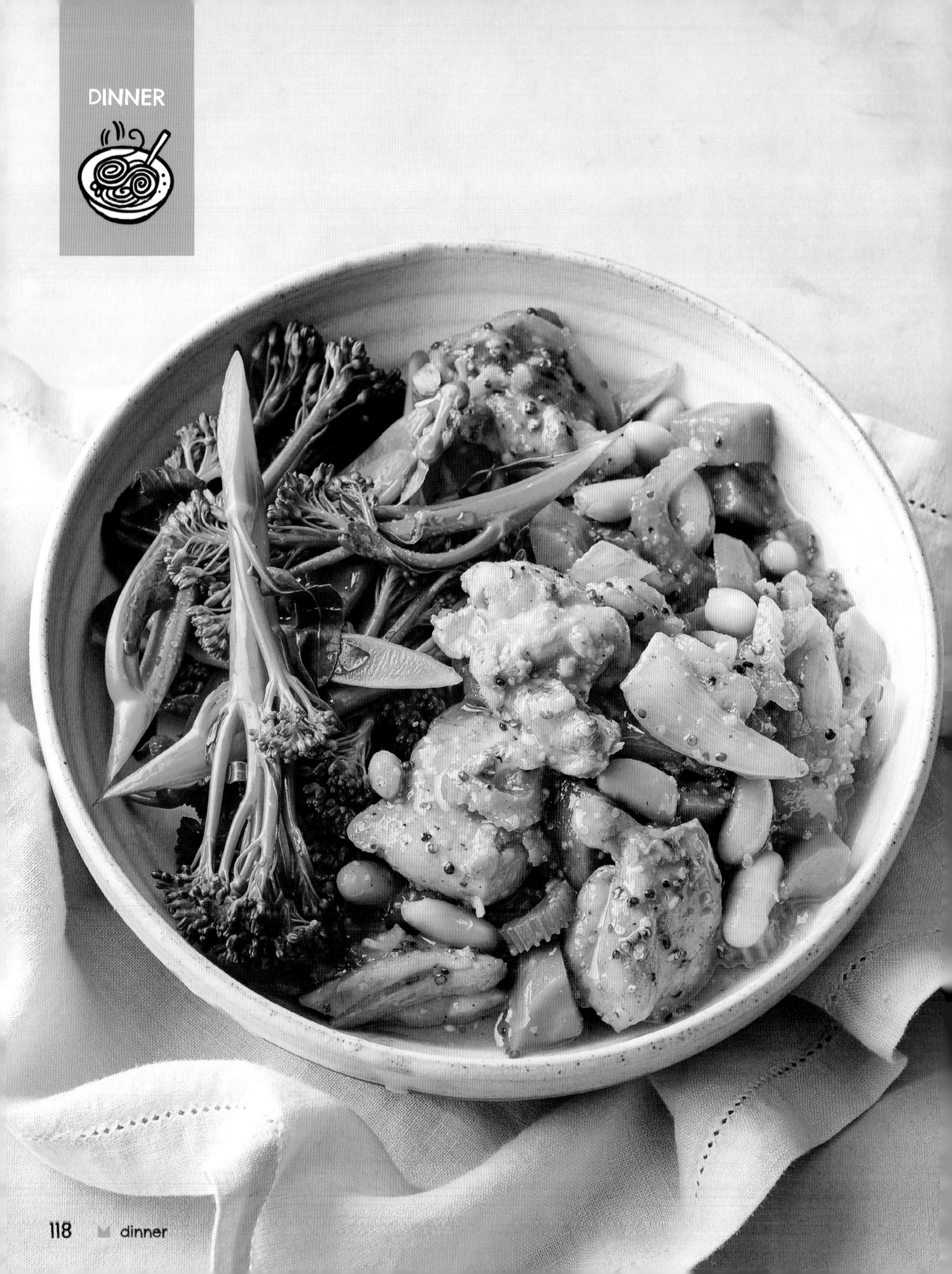

healthy apricot
CHICKEN

EF DF NF SF GF SBF FSF

We've brought traditional apricot chicken into the 2020s with this nutritious, reduced-fat and high-fibre recipe.

serves 4   prep 20 mins   cook 1 hour 5 mins

ingredients

2 tsp olive oil
600g skinless chicken thigh fillets, fat trimmed, cut into 3cm pieces
1 large brown onion, halved, thinly sliced
2 celery sticks, thinly sliced
2 carrots, peeled, cut into chunks
2 garlic cloves, crushed
1 tbs wholegrain mustard
125ml (½ cup) gluten-free chicken stock
250ml (1 cup) apricot nectar
35g (¼ cup) chopped dried apricots
400g can cannellini beans, rinsed, drained
Steamed snow peas and broccolini, to serve

1 Preheat oven to 170°C/150°C fan forced. Heat half the oil in a large flameproof casserole dish over high heat. In 2 batches, add chicken and cook for 1-2 minutes each side or until golden. Transfer to a plate.

2 Heat the remaining oil in the dish over medium heat. Add the onion, celery and carrot. Cook, stirring, for 5 minutes or until softened. Add the garlic and cook, stirring, for 30 seconds or until aromatic. Return chicken to the dish. Stir in the mustard, stock, apricot nectar and dried apricots. Bring to the boil.

3 Cover dish and bake for 40 minutes, adding the cannellini beans for the last 10 minutes of cooking time. Serve with the steamed greens.

PER SERVE 29.7g protein, 8.9g fat (2.3g saturated fat), 29.1g carb, 11.4g dietary fibre, 343 Cals (1432kJ)

make it your way

MUSTARD FREE Omit the wholegrain mustard if you have a mustard allergy and add 2 tsp horseradish in its place.

vegan zucchini
FRITTERS

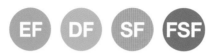

Family favourite zucchini fritters just went vegan!
With no egg or dairy, they're still packed with flavour
and perfect for midweek meals.

makes 8   prep 15 mins (+ standing & 20 mins soaking)   cook 10 mins

ingredients

600g (about 4) zucchini
1½ tbs flaxseed meal
2 tsp olive oil, plus extra,
    to shallow-fry and serve
3 green shallots, thinly sliced
2 garlic cloves, finely chopped
55g (½ cup) finely grated
    vegan cheese
75g (½ cup) self-raising flour
Pinch cayenne pepper
Halved cherry truss tomatoes,
    fresh mint leaves and thinly
    sliced red onion, to serve

1 Coarsely grate the zucchini. Transfer to a colander. Season and toss to combine. Set aside for 5 minutes. Take handfuls of zucchini and squeeze out as much liquid as possible. Transfer to a large bowl.

2 Meanwhile, place flaxseed and 80ml (⅓ cup) water in a small bowl. Stir to combine. Set aside to soak for 20 minutes.

3 Heat the oil in a frying pan over high heat. Add the shallot and garlic. Cook, stirring, for 2 minutes or until softened. Add to zucchini. Add flaxseed mixture and cheese. Sift in flour and cayenne. Mix to combine.

4 Pour enough oil in a large non-stick frying pan to come 3mm up the side. Place over medium heat. In batches, drop four ¼ cups of mixture into the oil and quickly spread to form approx. 8cm rounds. Cook, turning halfway, for 3 minutes or until golden and cooked through. Transfer to a plate lined with paper towel. Season and serve with the tomato, mint and onion, and a drizzle of olive oil.

PER SERVE 2.8g protein, 10.9g fat (2.7g saturated fat), 11.6g carb, 3.2g dietary fibre, 161 Cals (672kJ)

make it your way

NUT & SOY FREE Ensure the cheese is nut- and soy-free, if required.
GLUTEN FREE Use gluten-free self-raising flour and cheese.

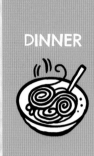

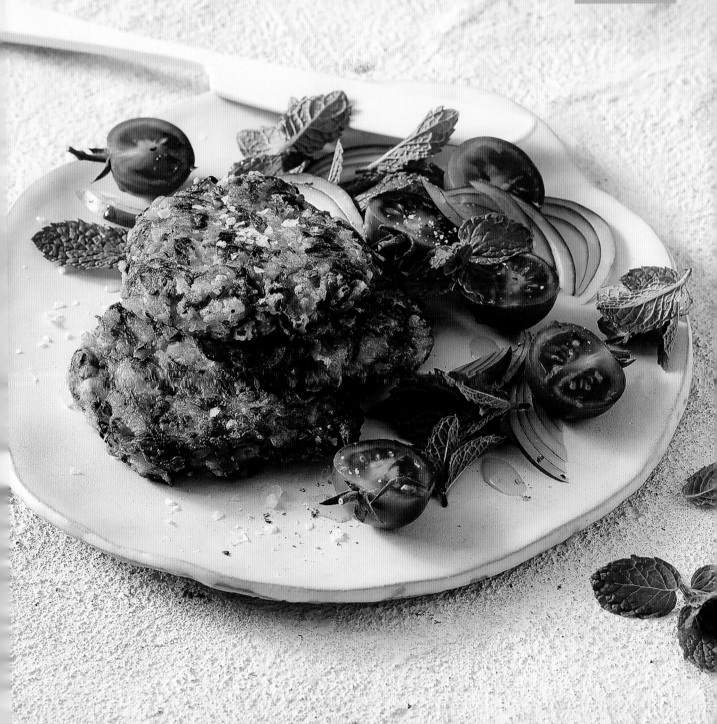

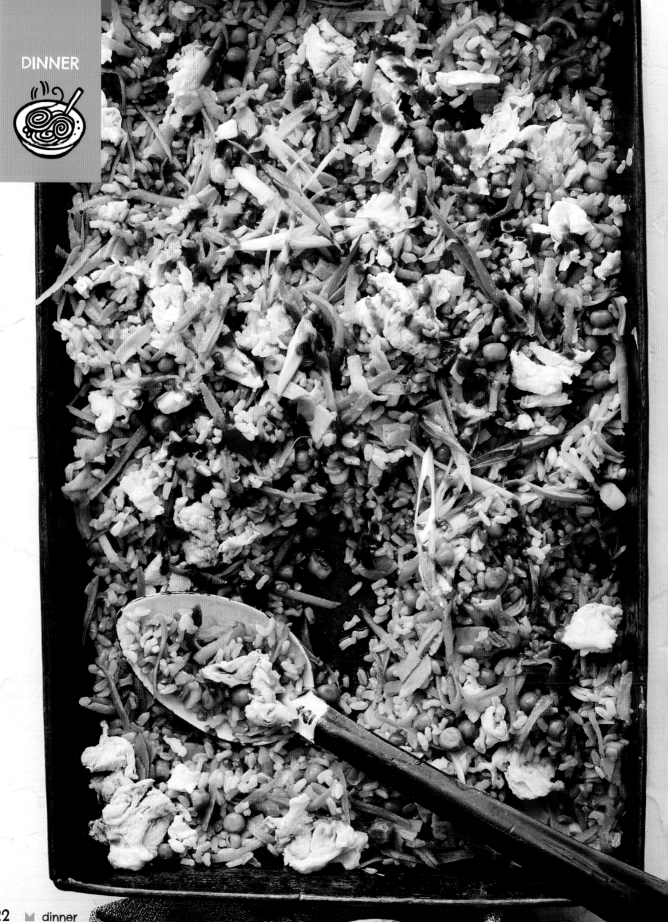

one-pan baked
FRIED RICE

There's no need for take away when you can cook this healthier fried rice in just one pan in the oven.

serves 4   prep 15 mins   cook 1 hour 5 mins

ingredients

300g (1½ cups) brown rice
2 garlic cloves, crushed
2 tsp grated fresh ginger
625ml (2½ cups) boiling water
2 tsp vegetable oil
2 carrots, peeled,
   coarsely grated
150g (1 cup) frozen peas
100g 97% fat-free, gluten-free
   sliced ham, chopped
3 green shallots, white and pale
   green section thinly sliced
   (green tops reserved)
2 tbs gluten-free soy or tamari
   sauce, plus extra, to serve
3 eggs
Sriracha chilli sauce, to serve

1   Preheat oven to 200°C/180°C fan forced. Place the rice in a 30 x 20cm (base size) baking dish. Add the garlic and ginger. Pour in the water and oil. Stir to combine. Cover the dish tightly with foil and bake for 45 minutes.

2   Carefully uncover the dish and stir in the carrot, peas, ham, white and pale green shallot, and the soy sauce. Re-cover with foil and cook for 10 minutes.

3   Remove and discard foil. Make 3 indentations in the rice mixture and break an egg into each. Use a fork to lightly whisk each egg without mixing into the rice. Return to the oven and cook, uncovered, for 7 minutes or until the egg is set.

4   Use a small sharp knife to coarsely chop the egg in the dish. Stir to combine. Diagonally slice the reserved shallot tops and sprinkle over the rice mixture. Serve drizzled with sriracha and extra soy sauce.

PER SERVE 17.8g protein, 8.8g fat (1.9g saturated fat), 62.8g carb, 8g dietary fibre, 419 Cals (1750kJ)

make it your way

SOY FREE Replace the soy sauce with coconut aminos sauce.
SWAP Substitute the ham with shredded roast chicken breast.

gluten-free prosciutto
PIZZA

Making your own gluten-free pizza dough is easy, and our simple selection of savoury toppings makes pizza nights a winner.

serves 4   prep 20 mins   cook 20 mins

ingredients

140g (1⅓ cups) mozzarella,
    coarsely grated, plus extra
    40g (⅓ cup), sliced
55g (½ cup) almond meal
2 tbs cream cheese
1 egg
80ml (⅓ cup) tomato
    pasta sauce
4 thin slices prosciutto
Fresh basil leaves, to serve

1 Place the grated mozzarella, almond meal and cream cheese in a microwave-safe bowl. Microwave for 1 minute, stirring halfway, or until melted and combined. Quickly add the egg and beat vigorously with a wooden spoon until combined.

2 Preheat oven to 200°C/180°C fan forced. Place the 'dough' between 2 pieces of baking paper and roll to line a 32cm pizza tray. Remove the top piece of baking paper and slide the dough with the bottom piece of baking paper onto the pizza tray. Prick with a fork. Bake for 10 minutes or until puffed and golden.

3 Flip over the pizza, remove the paper and cook for a further 5 minutes or until the top is golden. Spread lightly with tomato pasta sauce and top with extra sliced mozzarella. Bake for 3-4 minutes or until cheese is melted. Drape with prosciutto. Scatter with basil leaves, to serve.

PER SERVE 21g protein, 26.3g fat (10.7g saturated fat), 2.3g carb, 1.7g dietary fibre, 332 Cals (1386kJ)

make it your way
MEAT FREE Swap the prosciutto for sliced roma tomato and thinly sliced button mushrooms and red onion. Sprinkle the mozzarella on top.

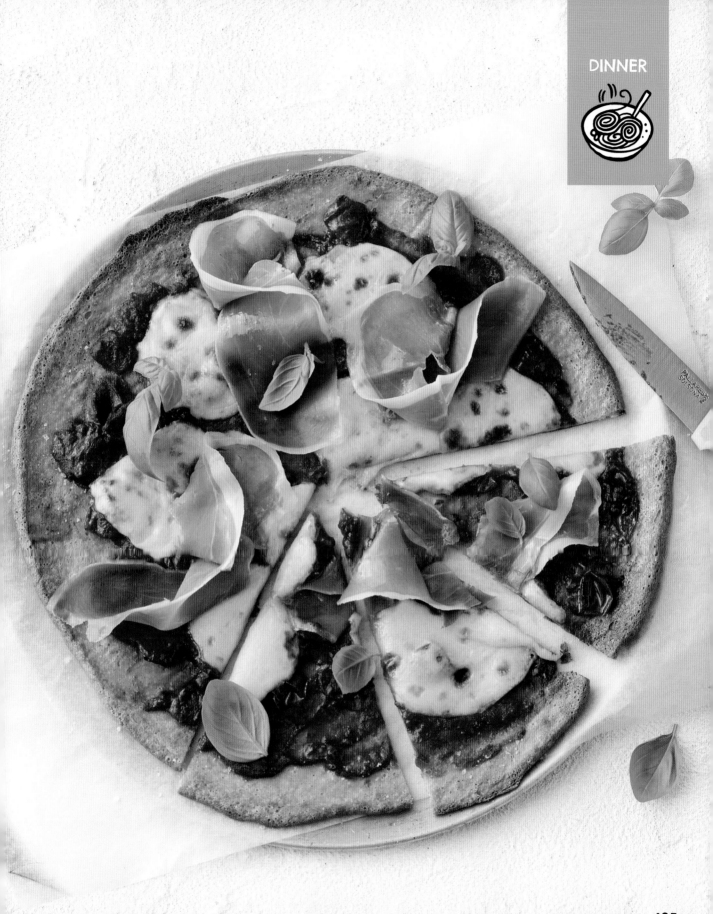

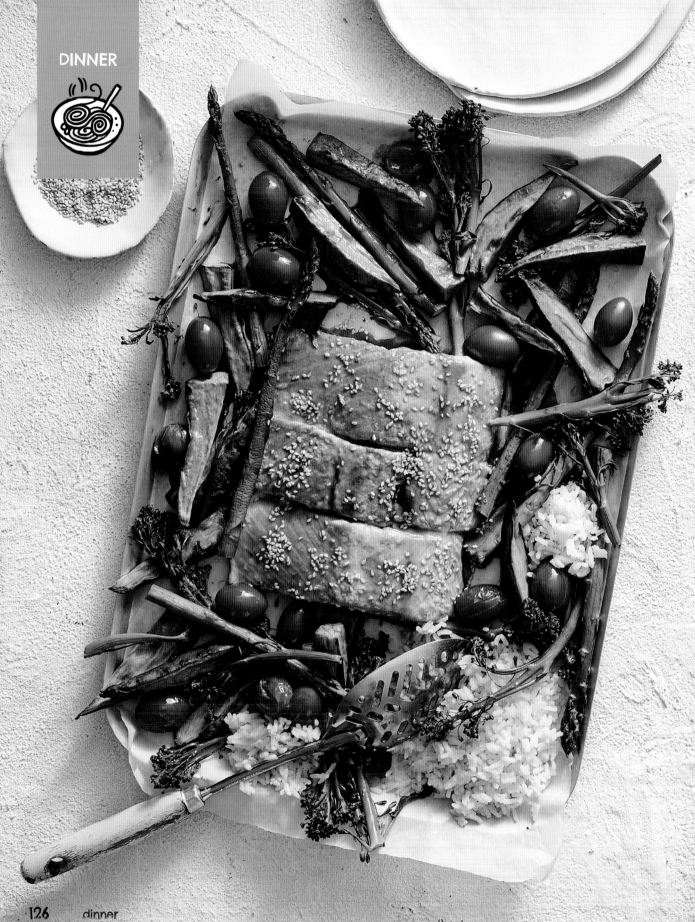

sticky japanese salmon
TRAY BAKE

An easy one-pan dinner loaded with sweet potato, tomato and broccolini, and drizzled in a flavour-packed dressing.

serves 4   prep 10 mins   cook 45 mins

ingredients

500g small sweet potatoes,
   cut into wedges
2 tbs mirin
2 tbs maple syrup
2 tbs gluten-free soy sauce
1 tbs fresh lime juice
4 skinless salmon fillets
1 bunch asparagus, trimmed,
   halved lengthways if thick
1 bunch broccolini, trimmed
200g punnet grape tomatoes
2 tsp toasted sesame seeds
Steamed white rice, to serve

1 Preheat oven to 200°C/180°C fan forced. Line a large baking tray with baking paper. Arrange the sweet potato wedges on the prepared tray. Spray with olive oil. Bake for 30 minutes or until tender.

2 Meanwhile, bring the mirin, maple syrup and soy sauce to the boil in a small saucepan over medium heat. Simmer for 3-5 minutes or until reduced by half. Transfer to a heatproof bowl and set aside, stirring occasionally, until slightly cooled. Stir in the lime juice.

3 Move the sweet potato to the tray edges and arrange the salmon in the centre. Drizzle one-third of the mirin mixture over the salmon. Arrange the asparagus, broccolini and tomatoes around the salmon.

4 Bake, drizzling salmon with remaining mirin mixture every 5 minutes, for 15 minutes. Sprinkle with sesame seeds. Serve with the rice.

PER SERVE 39.3g protein, 26.4g fat (5.8g saturated fat), 64.1g carb, 7.1g dietary fibre, 672 Cals (2811kJ)

make it your way

SESAME FREE Simply omit the sesame seeds or use flaxseeds instead.
SOY FREE Swap the soy sauce for coconut aminos sauce.

beef + pumpkin CURRY

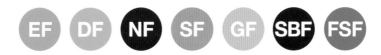

Sometimes you just need the comfort of a hearty curry. Sit down to this healthier take on a classic. It's sure to be a clean-plate hit with everyone at the table.

serves 4   prep 15 mins   cook 2 hours 15 mins

ingredients

2 garlic cloves, crushed

2 tsp fresh ginger, grated

1 tsp each of ground turmeric, coriander and cumin

2 long fresh red chillies, deseeded, chopped

2 red onions, finely chopped

500g lean beef blade steak

2 tsp olive oil

400g can crushed tomatoes

250ml (1 cup) salt-reduced, gluten-free beef stock

300g peeled pumpkin, chopped

1 large zucchini, chopped

60ml (¼ cup) reduced-fat coconut milk

120g baby spinach

Fresh coriander sprigs and steamed rice, to serve

1 Place the garlic, ginger, turmeric, coriander, cumin, chilli and half the onion in a food processor. Process until a coarse paste forms.

2 Trim fat from the beef and cut into 3cm pieces. Heat 1 tsp oil in a large saucepan over high heat. Cook the beef, in 2 batches, stirring, for 2-3 minutes or until browned. Transfer to a plate.

3 Heat the remaining oil in the pan over medium heat. Add remaining onion and cook, stirring, for 3-4 minutes or until softened. Add spice paste and stir for 2 minutes or until aromatic.

4 Return beef to the pan with the tomato and stock. Cover and bring to the boil over medium heat. Reduce heat to low and simmer for 1½ hours. Add the pumpkin. Simmer, uncovered, for 15 minutes. Add zucchini and 2 tbs coconut milk. Simmer for 5 minutes or until pumpkin is tender. Season. Stir through the spinach. Drizzle with remaining 1 tbs coconut milk. Top with coriander. Serve with rice.

PER SERVE 35g protein, 10g fat (3g saturated fat), 44g carb, 8g dietary fibre, 430 Cals (1801kJ)

make it your way

FREEZE IT Place the curry an airtight container and freeze for up to 2 months. Thaw in the fridge, then reheat to serve on a busy night.

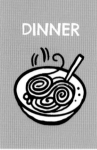
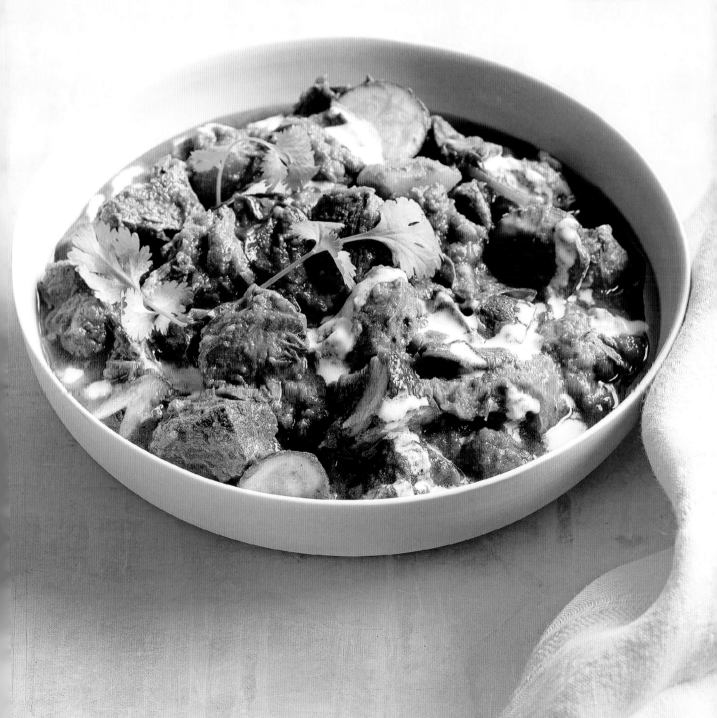

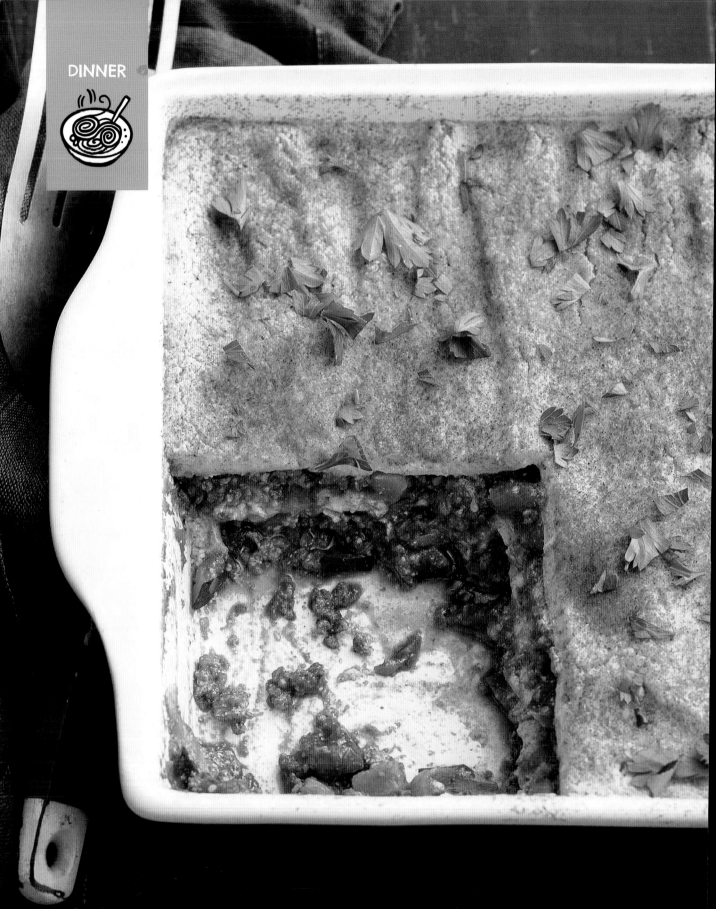

dairy-free
LASAGNE

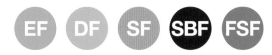

This delicious lasagne has a better-for-you version of bechamel to take your enjoyment to the next level. It's not traditional but it hits the spot!

serves 6   prep 50 mins (+ standing)   cook 1½ hours

ingredients

290g (2 cups) unsalted cashews
250ml (1 cup) vegetable stock
80ml (⅓ cup) almond milk
1 tbs extra virgin olive oil
1 brown onion, finely chopped
2 garlic cloves, crushed
1 carrot, peeled, finely chopped
1 celery stalk, finely chopped
1 zucchini, finely chopped
½ eggplant, finely chopped
750g beef mince
2 x 400g cans crushed tomatoes
140g (½ cup) tomato paste
8 fresh lasagne sheets
½ tsp sweet paprika
Chopped fresh continental
   parsley leaves, to serve

1. Place cashews in a heatproof bowl. Cover with boiling water. Stand for 10 minutes. Drain. Place in a food processor with half the stock. Process until smooth. Add milk. Process until combined. Season.

2. Preheat oven to 180°C/160°C fan forced. Grease a 7cm-deep, 23 x 30cm (12 cup) ovenproof dish. Heat the oil in a large saucepan over medium-high heat. Add onion, garlic, carrot and celery. Cook, stirring, for 5 minutes or until softened. Add zucchini and eggplant. Cook, stirring, for 5 minutes or until softened. Add beef. Cook, breaking up lumps with a wooden spoon, for 5 minutes or until browned. Stir in tomato, tomato paste and remaining stock. Reduce heat to low. Simmer, stirring occasionally, for 20 minutes or until sauce thickens. Season.

3. Spread half the beef mixture in prepared dish. Top with 4 lasagne sheets, trimming to fit. Spread with half the cashew mixture. Repeat layers.

4. Cover dish with baking paper, then foil. Bake for 45 minutes. Sprinkle with paprika. Bake, uncovered, for 10 minutes or until tender and top is golden. Stand for 10 minutes. Sprinkle with parsley, to serve.

PER SERVE 46.6g protein, 39.8g fat (9.3g saturated fat), 51.9 carb, 9g dietary fibre, 771 Cals (3227kJ)

make it your way

GLUTEN FREE Use gluten-free lasagne sheets. BOOST Sprinkle the lasagne with coconut cheese at the end of step 4, before baking.

loaded vegetarian NACHOS

Mexican Mondays get a makeover with this vegie-packed version of nachos. Adjust the heat to match your tolerance.

serves 4   prep 20 mins   cook 20 mins

ingredients

6 x 28g corn tortillas
2 tsp olive oil
1 red onion, finely chopped
2 garlic cloves, crushed
1 long fresh red chilli,
    finely chopped
1 tsp ground cumin
1 tsp smoked paprika,
    plus extra, to sprinkle
1 large red capsicum,
    deseeded, chopped
1 large zucchini, chopped
400g can black beans,
    rinsed, drained
400g can diced tomatoes
150g green beans, chopped
130g (½ cup) natural yoghurt
Fresh coriander leaves and
    lime wedges, to serve

1 Preheat oven to 180°C/160°C fan forced. Line 2 large baking trays with baking paper. Cut each tortilla into 12 wedges. Place on the prepared trays and lightly spray with olive oil. Bake, turning once, for 12-15 minutes or until golden and crisp. Set aside.

2 Meanwhile, heat the oil in a large saucepan over medium heat. Add the onion and garlic. Cook, stirring, for 5 minutes or until softened. Add the chilli, cumin and paprika. Cook, stirring, for 1 minute or until aromatic. Add the capsicum and zucchini. Cook, stirring, for 1 minute or until softened slightly.

3 Add black beans, tomato and 80ml (⅓ cup) water to the pan. Bring to the boil. Reduce heat to low. Simmer for 10 minutes or until thickened. Add green beans. Simmer for 2 minutes or until just tender.

4 Arrange the tortilla wedges and bean mixture on serving plates. Serve with yoghurt, coriander, lime wedges and a sprinkle of paprika.

PER SERVE 14g protein, 8.8g fat (2.4g saturated fat), 41.2g carb, 13.2g dietary fibre, 331 Cals (1384kJ)

make it your way

DAIRY FREE Use a plant-based yoghurt. BEAT THE HEAT Remove and discard the seeds from the chilli before finely chopping.

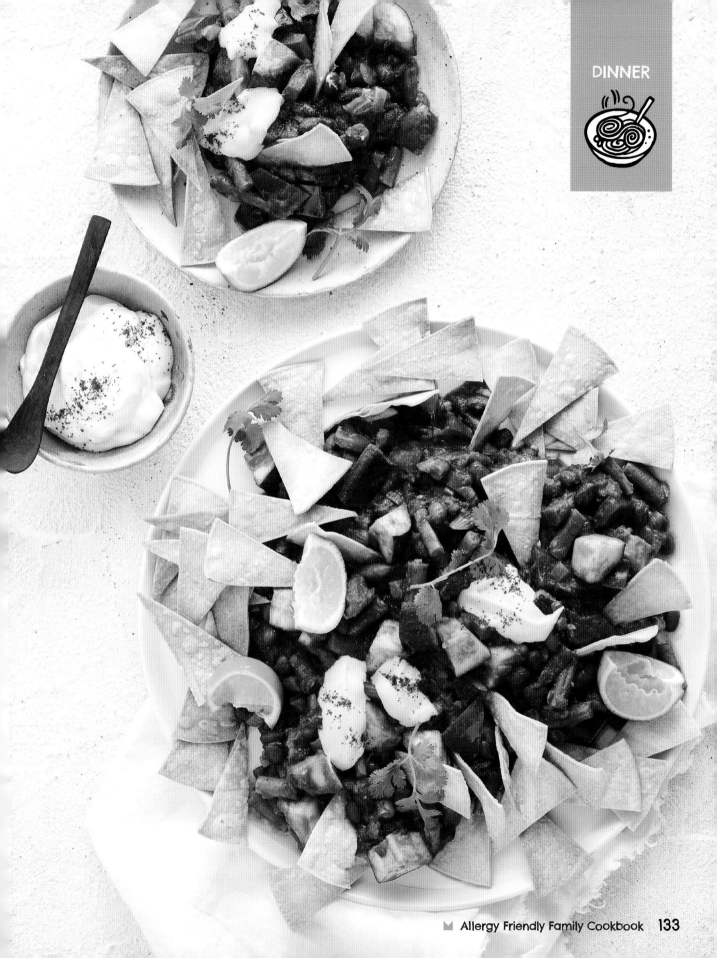

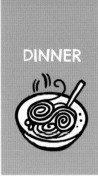
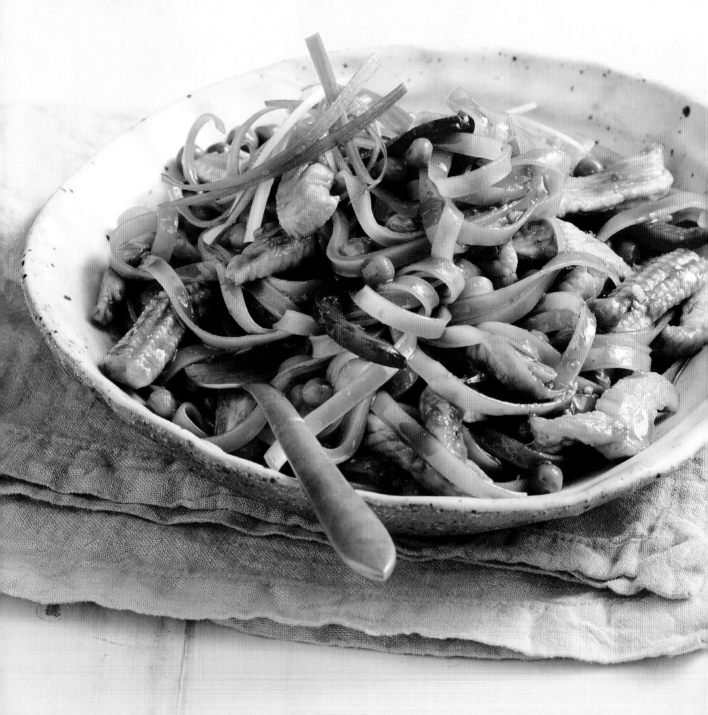

honey chicken noodle
STIR-FRY

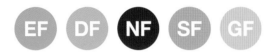

Great for weeknights, this quick and easy stir-fry has a delicious honey, soy and oyster sauce that the whole family will love.

serves 4   prep 15 mins (+ 10 mins soaking)   cook 15 mins

ingredients

200g dried rice stick noodles
60ml (¼ cup) gluten-free
   soy or tamari sauce
2 tbs gluten-free oyster sauce
2 tbs honey
1½ tbs extra virgin olive oil
500g chicken breast
   stir-fry pieces
3 tsp finely chopped ginger
2 garlic cloves, crushed
1 red capsicum, deseeded,
   chopped
115g pkt baby corn, halved
150g (1 cup) frozen peas
Green shallots, thinly sliced,
   to serve

1 Place the noodles in a heatproof bowl. Cover with boiling water and set aside for 10 minutes to soak. Drain. Combine the soy sauce, oyster sauce and honey in a jug.

2 Heat 1 tbs oil in a wok over high heat. Add the chicken and cook for 3 minutes. Turn pieces over and cook for a further 3 minutes or until golden. Use tongs to transfer to a plate. Set aside.

3 Heat the remaining oil in the wok. Add the ginger and garlic. Cook, stirring, for 1 minute or until aromatic. Add capsicum and corn. Cook, stirring, for 1 minute or until starting to brown. Add 2 tbs water. Cook, stirring, for 3 minutes or until the water evaporates and the vegies are tender.

4 Add the honey mixture, chicken, drained noodles and peas to the wok. Use tongs to toss to combine. Serve sprinkled with shallot.

PER SERVE 36.6g protein, 9.9g fat (2.2g saturated fat), 61.6g carb, 6.3g dietary fibre, 491 Cals (2054kJ)

make it your way

FISH & SHELLFISH FREE Use vegan soy sauce or tamari (contains soy), and swap the oyster sauce for vegetarian oyster sauce.

slow-cooked beef
DUMP DINNER

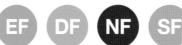 EF DF NF SF 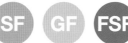 GF FSF

This good old-fashioned beef casserole involves you 'dumping' all the ingredients into the slow cooker and then forgetting about it until dinnertime. Enjoy!

serves 4   prep 10 mins   cook 8 hours

ingredients

1kg gravy beef, cut into chunks
2 tbs gluten-free traditional
   gravy powder
1 tbs gluten-free plain flour
500g baby potatoes, halved
200g button mushrooms, halved
2 carrots, peeled, chopped
6 French shallots, peeled,
   halved
125ml (½ cup) gluten-free
   beef stock
400g can diced tomatoes
225g jar tomato chutney
Steamed green vegetables,
   to serve (optional)

1 Place the beef in a slow cooker. Add the gravy powder and plain flour, and toss to coat the beef.

2 Toss the potato, mushroom, carrot and shallot into the slow cooker. Pour over the stock, then add the tomato and chutney.

3 Cover slow cooker with the lid. Cook on High for 8 hours or until the beef is very tender. Serve with the vegetables, if desired.

PER SERVE 54.9g protein, 11.6g fat (4.2g saturated fat), 53.9g carb, 6.8g dietary fibre, 559 Cals (2338kJ)

make it your way

SWAP IT Instead of gravy beef, try beef chuck steak, cut into pieces.
BOOST Toss in some chopped swede or turnip in step 2, if you like.

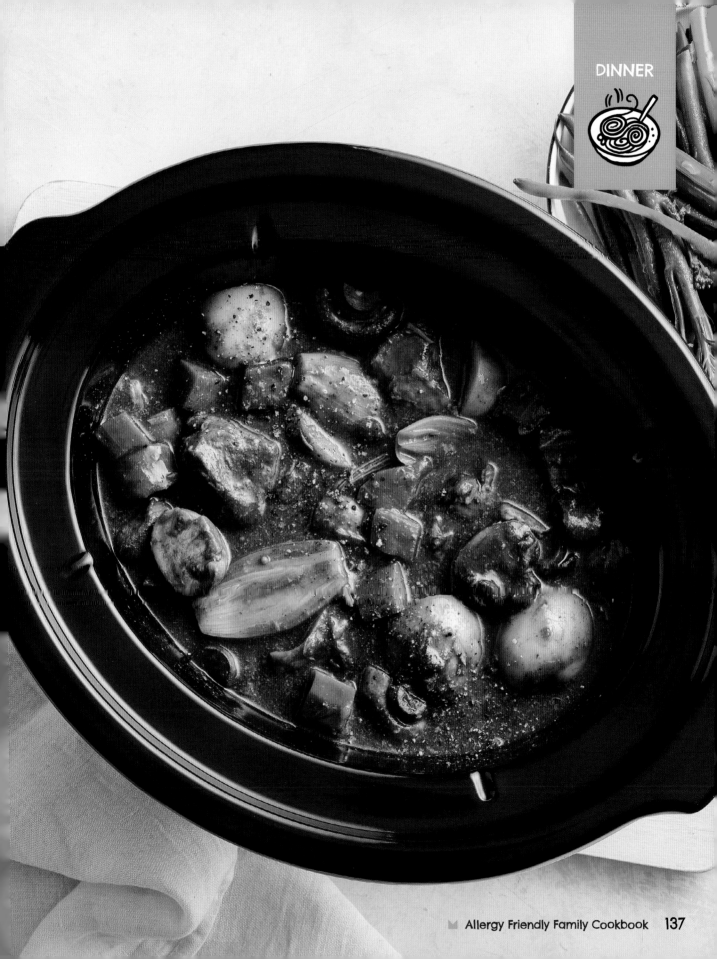

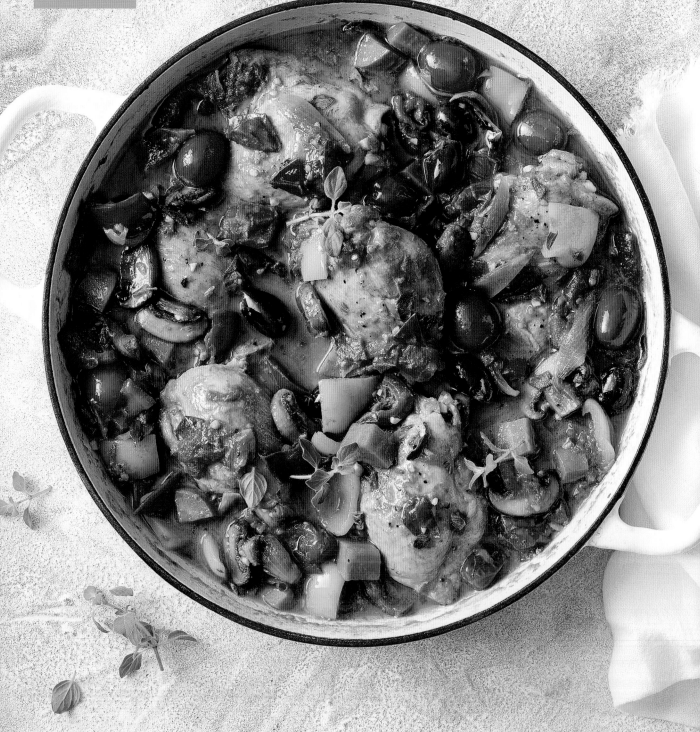

so good chicken
CACCIATORE

Who doesn't love chicken cacciatore? And this healthier version lives up to it's 'so good' name in both nutrition and flavour. Buon appetito!

serves 6   prep 25 mins   cook 1 hour 5 mins

ingredients

1.1kg (about 6) chicken thigh cutlets, skin removed
2 tbs olive oil
200g Swiss brown mushrooms, sliced
1 red onion, thinly sliced
4 tomatoes, chopped
4 garlic cloves, chopped
1 red capsicum, deseeded, chopped
1 yellow capsicum, deseeded, chopped
1 carrot, peeled, chopped
125ml (½ cup) white wine
250ml (1 cup) gluten-free chicken stock
200g punnet grape tomatoes
60g (¼ cup) pitted kalamata olives
2 tbs chopped fresh oregano, plus extra sprigs, to serve

1 Season the chicken cutlets well. Heat 1 tbs olive oil in a large non-stick frying pan over medium-high heat. Add chicken and cook for 2-3 minutes each side or until browned all over. Transfer to a plate.

2 Add the mushroom to the pan and reduce heat to medium. Cook, stirring, for 3-4 minutes or until softened. Transfer to a bowl. Add the remaining 1 tbs oil to the pan. Add the onion and cook, stirring, for 2-3 minutes or until just beginning to soften.

3 Add tomato and garlic to the pan. Cook, stirring, for 3-4 minutes or until softened. Add capsicum and carrot. Cook, stirring, for 2 minutes. Add wine. Simmer for 5 minutes or until liquid reduces by half.

4 Return chicken and mushroom to the pan. Add stock, tomatoes and olives. Bring to the boil. Reduce heat to low. Cover and simmer for 20 minutes. Uncover and simmer for a further 20 minutes or until the sauce is thickened. Stir in the oregano. Season. Serve scattered with extra oregano sprigs.

PER SERVE 33g protein, 22g fat (5g saturated fat), 9g carb, 6g dietary fibre, 400 Cals (1675kJ)

make it your way

BOOST Serve with thick slices of crusty gluten- and soy-free bread.
SWAP Use cherry tomatoes instead of grape tomatoes, if you like.

one-pot mexican
BEEF MINCE

This is Mexican fare with a veg hit. The kids will love it, and the parents will feel good knowing the kids are getting a good dose of vegies. It's win win!

serves 4   prep 10 mins   cook 25 mins

ingredients

2 tsp extra virgin olive oil
1 red onion, halved, sliced
1 red and 1 green capsicum, deseeded, chopped
2 garlic cloves, crushed
2 tsp smoked paprika
2 tsp dried oregano
1 tsp ground cumin
500g lean beef mince
2 tbs no-added-salt tomato paste
250ml (1 cup) gluten-free beef stock
250g pkt 2-minute brown & wild rice
Light sour cream, chopped avocado, fresh coriander sprigs, sliced red chilli and lime halves, to serve

1 Heat the oil in large frying pan over medium-high heat. Add the onion and capsicum. Cook, stirring occasionally, for 5 minutes or until starting to soften. Add the garlic, paprika, oregano and cumin. Cook, stirring, for 30 seconds or until aromatic. Add the beef. Cook, breaking up lumps with a wooden spoon, for 6-8 minutes or until beef is browned.

2 Add the tomato paste, stock and 125ml (½ cup) water to the pan. Bring to a simmer. Stir in the rice. Reduce heat to medium-low. Cook, uncovered, for 8-10 minutes or until liquid is absorbed. Top with sour cream, avocado, coriander and chilli. Serve with lime halves.

PER SERVE 36.1g protein, 18.3g fat (5.6g saturated fat), 28.6g carb, 10.4g dietary fibre, 444 Cals (1856kJ)

make it your way

DAIRY FREE Use dairy-free sour cream. SWAP Omit the rice and serve the beef mixture over corn chips as a tasty nacho feast.

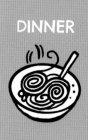

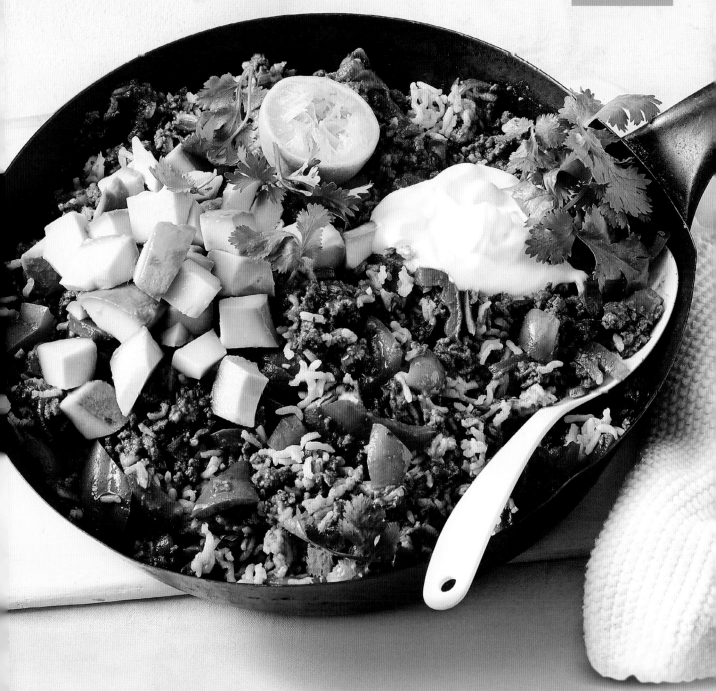

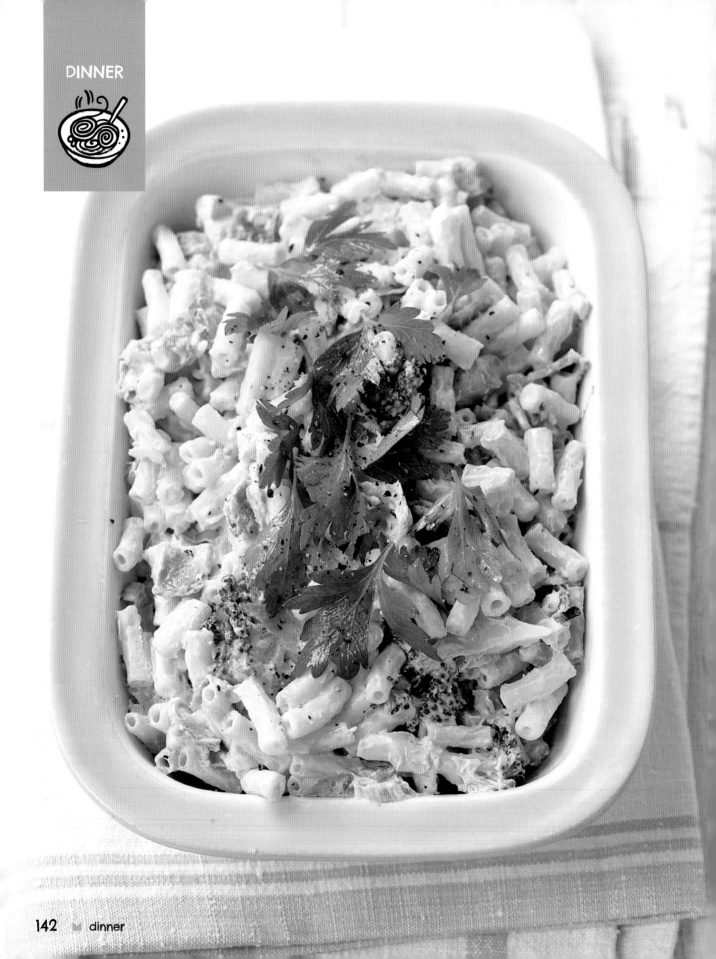

dairy-free macaroni
CHEESE

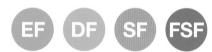

Nobody should miss out on this weeknight staple. That's why you need to bookmark this dairy-free version — it's a keeper!

serves 4   prep 10 mins   cook 35 mins

ingredients

250g (2½ cups) dried
   macaroni pasta
250g broccoli, trimmed, cut
   into small florets
20g Nuttelex spread
2 tbs plain flour
500ml (2 cups) reduced-fat
   soy milk
105g (1¼ cups) plant-based
   cheddar, grated
100g sliced leg ham, chopped
4 green shallots, trimmed,
   thinly sliced
Salad leaves and fresh
   continental parsley leaves,
   to serve

1 Preheat oven to 180°C/160°C fan forced. Grease a 6-cup baking dish. Cook the pasta in a large saucepan of salted boiling water following packet directions or until al dente, adding broccoli for the last 2 minutes of cooking time. Drain well. Transfer to a large bowl.

2 Meanwhile, melt the spread in a saucepan over medium heat. Add the flour. Cook, stirring, for 2 minutes or until bubbling. Gradually add milk, whisking constantly. Bring to the boil. Cook, whisking, for 5 minutes or until thickened. Remove from the heat. Stir in the cheddar. Season with pepper.

3 Add the sauce, ham and shallot to the pasta. Stir to combine. Spoon into prepared baking dish. Bake for 15-20 minutes or until golden and bubbling. Serve with salad leaves and scattered with parsley.

PER SERVE 21.9g protein, 15.4g fat (2.8g saturated fat), 53.4g carb, 6g dietary fibre, 451 Cals (1889kJ)

make it your way NUT FREE Ensure cheese is nut free. GLUTEN FREE Use gluten-free macaroni and gluten-free plain flour. Also, ensure your leg ham is gluten free. SOY FREE Opt for soy-free milk and cheese.

lentil balls in roasted
TOMATO

EF NF SF GF SBF FSF

These vego lentil meatballs are cooked in a flavoursome cherry tomato sauce that's also low in calories.

serves 4   prep 25 mins   cook 50 mins

ingredients

750g cherry truss tomatoes,
    removed from the vine, halved
2 tsp fresh thyme leaves
6 garlic cloves, thinly sliced
1 tbs olive oil
1 onion, finely chopped
2 celery sticks, trimmed, diced
300g mushrooms, chopped
400g can lentils, rinsed, drained
¼ cup chopped fresh basil, plus
    basil sprigs, extra, to serve
90g (½ cup) microwave brown
    rice, warmed
2 tbs coconut flour
2 tsp finely grated lemon rind
2 tbs finely grated parmesan,
    plus extra 2 tbs, to serve
Rocket, to serve

1 Preheat oven to 180°C/160°C fan forced. Arrange tomato in a baking dish. Toss in thyme and half the garlic. Drizzle with 1 tsp oil. Season. Cover dish with foil. Bake for 40 minutes or until tomato softens.

2 Meanwhile, heat 1 tsp oil in a large non-stick frying pan over medium heat. Add onion and celery. Cook, stirring, for 3-4 minutes or until softened. Add mushroom and remaining garlic. Cook, stirring, for 4 minutes or until mushroom is golden. Set aside to cool.

3 Process lentils in a food processor until crumbs form. Add the onion mixture, basil, rice, flour, lemon rind and parmesan. Pulse to combine. Season. Use hands to roll tablespoonfuls of mixture into 24 balls.

4 Heat remaining 2 tsp oil in the frying pan over medium-high heat. Cook lentil balls, turning, for 3-4 minutes or until golden.

5 Add lentil balls to dish with the tomatoes. Bake, uncovered, for 10 minutes. Top with the extra basil and parmesan. Serve with rocket.

PER SERVE 14g protein, 8g fat (2g saturated fat), 30g carb, 11g dietary fibre, 278 Cals (1160kJ)

make it your way

GET AHEAD Bake tomato in step 1. Cool. Chill in fridge for up to 2 days.
DAIRY FREE Use dairy-free parmesan (may contain soy and nuts).

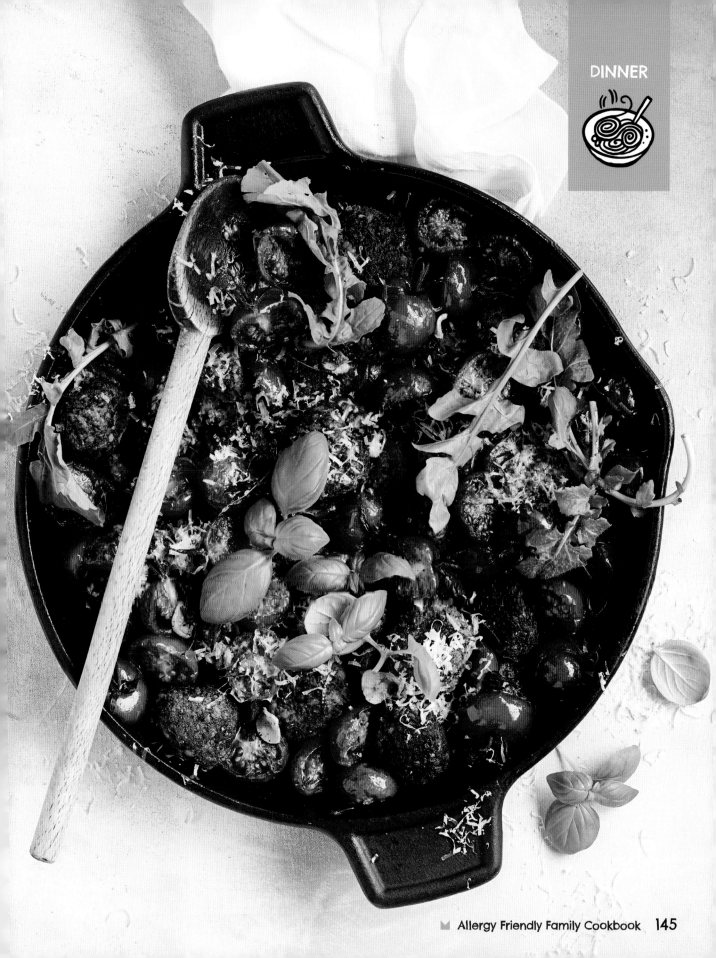

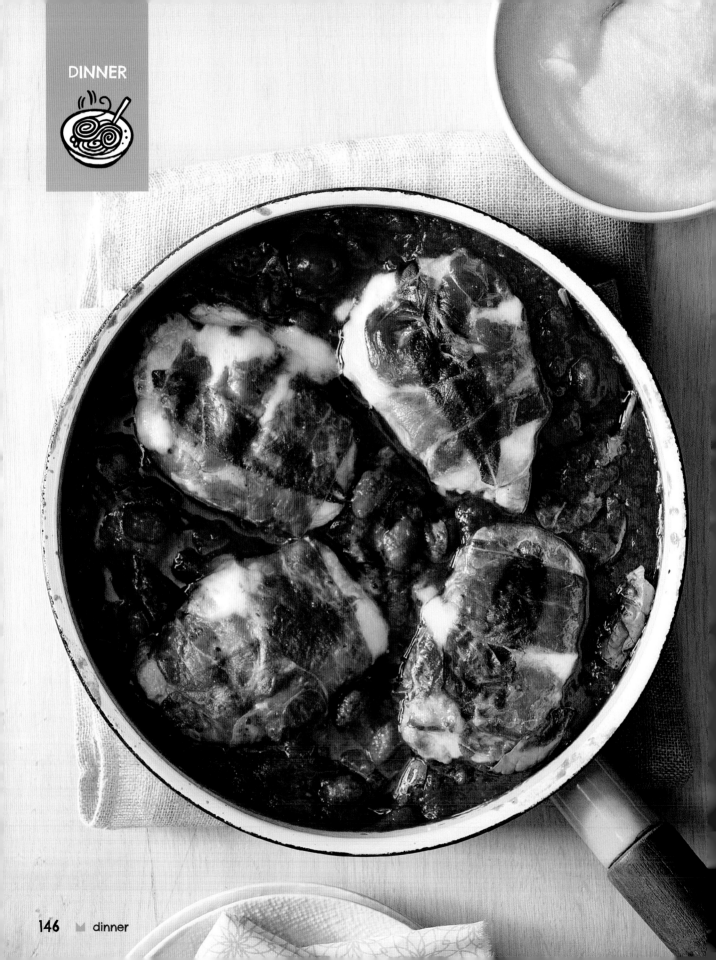

spicy borlotti bean
SALTIMBOCCA

This succulent pork wrapped in prosciutto has a gooey mozzarella centre that literally oozes in the mouth. Delish!

serves 4   prep 10 mins   cook 20 mins

ingredients

4 pork loin medallions
85g mozzarella, thinly sliced
4 large fresh sage leaves
4 slices prosciutto
1 tbs olive oil
420g jar arrabbiata pasta sauce
125ml (½ cup) gluten-free chicken stock
400g can borlotti beans, rinsed, drained
60g baby spinach leaves
Soft polenta, to serve

1 Preheat oven to 180°C/160°C fan forced. Top each pork medallion with a slice of mozzarella and a sage leaf. Wrap a slice of prosciutto right around the bundle to enclose.

2 Heat the oil in a large ovenproof frying pan over medium-high heat. Add wrapped pork and cook for 1 minute each side or until light golden. Transfer to a plate. Add pasta sauce and stock to the pan and bring to the boil. Season.

3 Remove from heat. Return pork to pan, sage side up. Bake for 10 minutes. Add borlotti beans and spinach. Cover and bake for 5 minutes or until spinach just wilts. Serve with the polenta.

PER SERVE 50.5g protein, 19.2g fat (6.7g saturated fat), 45g carb, 10.5g dietary fibre, 579 Cals (2422kJ)

make it your way

DAIRY FREE Use dairy-free mozzarella (may contain soy and nuts).
TRY Serve with baked potatoes and steamed greens instead of polenta.

eggplant + sweet
POTATO CURRY

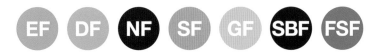

EF DF **NF** SF GF **SBF** FSF

"When more than one allergy abounds, it's dishes like this comforting curry that make eating a joy once again." ~ *Tegan Laird*

serves 4   prep 25 mins   cook 40 mins

ingredients

2 tbs coconut oil

1 brown onion, thinly sliced

1 garlic clove, crushed

1 tsp finely grated ginger

20 fresh curry leaves

1 quantity masala paste (see recipe, below right)

2 tbs soy-free tamarind puree

400ml can coconut milk

500ml (2 cups) gluten-free vegetable stock

400g (1 large) eggplant, chopped

300g sweet potato, chopped

1 zucchini, grated

1 carrot, grated

100g baby spinach leaves

200g (1 cup) basmati rice, steamed

Lime wedges, to serve

1 Heat the oil in a large saucepan over medium heat. Add the onion. Cook, stirring, for 5 minutes or until softened. Add garlic, ginger, curry leaves and masala paste. Cook, stirring, for 2 minutes or until aromatic.

2 Stir in the tamarind puree, coconut milk and stock. Bring to the boil. Add all vegetables apart from the spinach. Reduce heat to medium-low and simmer, uncovered, for 30 minutes or until vegetables are tender and the sauce is slightly thickened. Stir in the spinach. Serve curry with the rice and lime wedges for squeezing.

PER SERVE 11.7g protein, 34.5g fat (28g saturated fat), 68g carb, 12.6g dietary fibre, 648 Cals (2707kJ)

Masala paste Place 1 tbs coriander seeds, 2 tsp cumin seeds, and 1 tsp black peppercorns, in a frying pan over medium heat. Cook, stirring, for 1-2 minutes or until lightly toasted and aromatic. Transfer to a small food processor. Process until coarsely ground. Add 45g (½ cup) desiccated coconut and 2 tsp ground turmeric. Process until combined. Add the juice of 1 lime and 60ml (¼ cup) water. Process until a coarse paste forms. Set aside.

make it your way

FREEZE IT Freeze cooled curry in an airtight container for up to 2 months. Thaw in the fridge before reheating to serve.

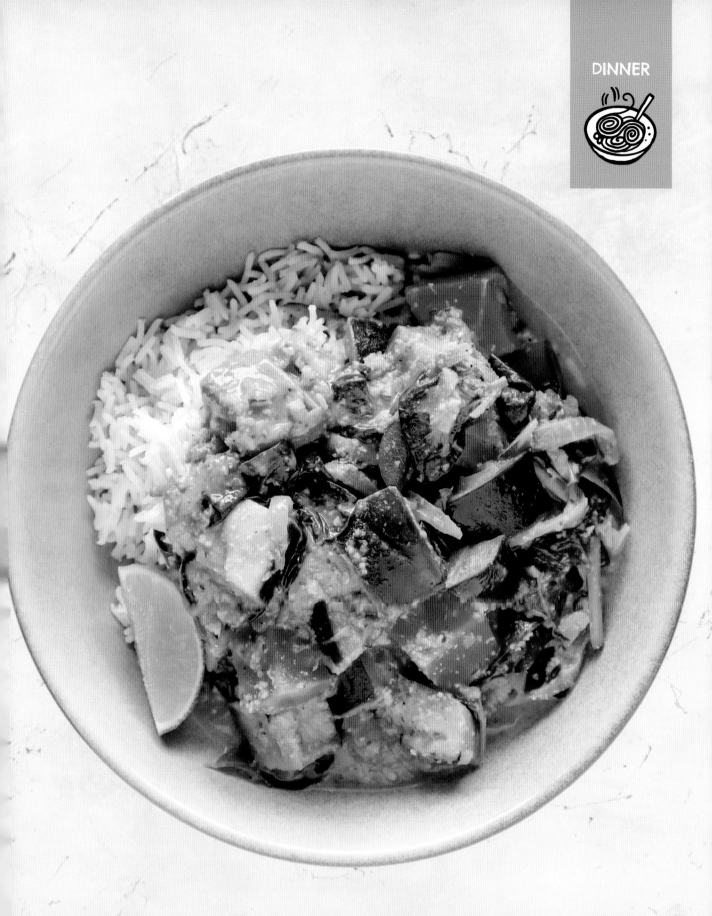

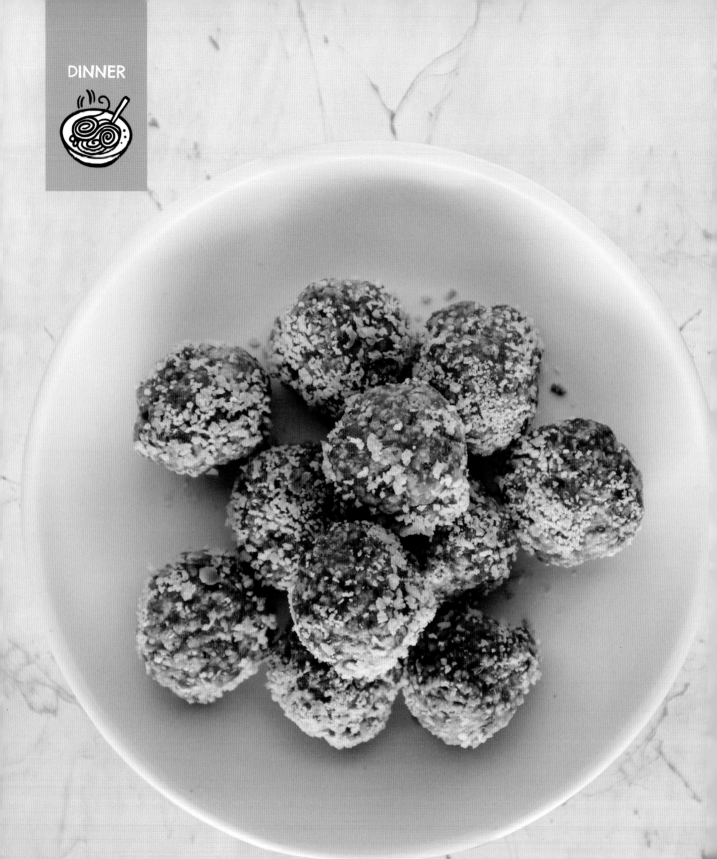

'dinosaur egg'
MEATBALLS

"As a toddler, Axel had critically low B12 and no interest in food. We started watching cooking shows in desperation and he loved Mary Berry. Her meatball recipe included egg and cheese (Ax has anaphylaxis to egg, dairy and nuts). I tried to come up with something similar and ended up with this recipe." ~ *Sarah MacFarlane*

makes 24   prep 20 mins   cook 30 mins

ingredients

420g can peas and carrots, drained
190g pkt panko breadcrumbs
1 tsp salt
1 tsp garlic powder
1 tsp ground paprika (optional)
500g lean pork mince
Vegetable oil, to coat

1 Preheat oven to 200°C/180°C fan forced. Place the vegetables in a large bowl. Use a stick blender to blend until mushy.

2 Reserve 25g (¼ cup) breadcrumbs. Add remaining breadcrumbs to the vegetables. Stir in the salt, garlic powder and paprika, if using. Add the mince and use a fork or clean hands to evenly combine. Roll slightly heaped tablespoonfuls of the mixture into 24 balls.

3 Stand a wire rack on a baking tray. Place a little oil in a small dish. Place reserved breadcrumbs on a small plate. In batches, toss balls in oil, then roll in reserved breadcrumbs to coat. Place on the wire rack.

4 Bake the meatballs for 30 minutes or until cooked through and golden brown all over. Serve warm.

PER MEATBALL 5.5g protein, 3.3g fat (1g saturated fat), 6.3g carb, 0.8g dietary fibre, 78 Cals (326kJ)

 make it your way

GLUTEN & SOY FREE Instead of panko, use gluten- and soy-free breadcrumbs. FREEZE IT Freeze uncooked meatballs for up to 1 month.

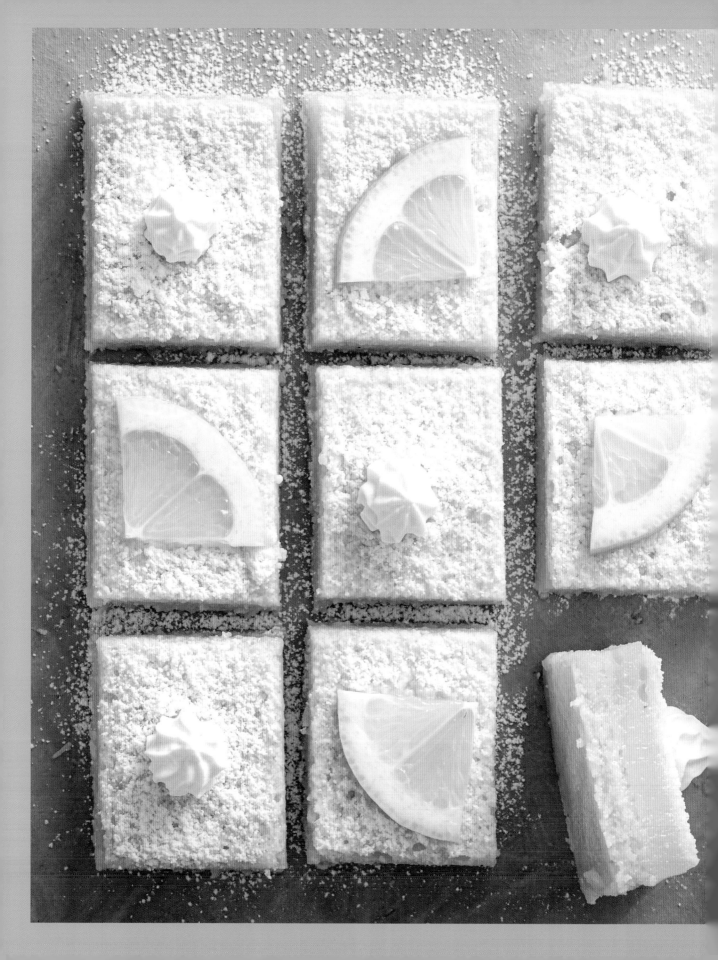

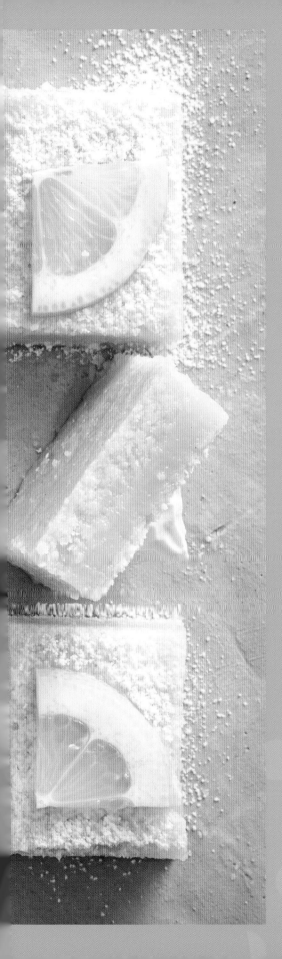

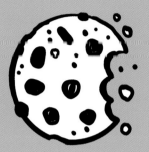

sweet treats

Turn to these pages when the bake sale calls for slices, bikkies, brownies and more.

easy jaffa
MARBLE LOAF

With sweet swirls of tangy orange and silky dark chocolate, the jaffa flavour really comes alive in this gluten-free treat.

serves 12   prep 25 mins (+ cooling)   cook 50 mins

ingredients

185ml (¾ cup) reduced-fat milk
125ml (½ cup) fresh orange
    juice, strained
1 tbs finely grated orange rind
100ml extra virgin olive oil
150g coconut sugar
2 eggs, lightly whisked
160g (1 cup) buckwheat flour
40g coconut flour
2 tbs almond meal
1 tsp gluten-free baking powder
½ tsp bicarbonate of soda
2 tbs 70% dark chocolate,
    coarsely chopped
30g (¼ cup) raw cacao, sifted

1 Preheat oven to 180°C/160°C fan forced. Grease the base and sides of a 9.5 x 19.5cm (base size) loaf pan and line with baking paper.

2 Place the milk, orange juice and rind, oil and sugar in a small saucepan over low heat. Cook, stirring, for 5 minutes or until sugar dissolves (mixture may curdle). Transfer to a bowl. Cool for 5 minutes.

3 Stir egg into the milk mixture. Reserve 40g (¼ cup) buckwheat flour. Add remaining buckwheat flour to the saucepan. Add coconut flour, almond meal, baking powder and bicarb. Stir until smooth. Transfer half the batter to a second bowl. Stir the chocolate and reserved buckwheat flour into 1 bowl. Stir cacao into remaining bowl.

4 Spoon half the batters, in random spoonfuls, into the prepared loaf pan. Use a butter knife to create a swirled effect. Repeat with remaining batters and butter knife. Bake for 45 minutes or until a skewer inserted in the centre comes out clean. Cool in pan for 10 minutes. Transfer to a wire rack to cool completely. Serve.

PER SERVE 3g protein, 11g fat (3g saturated fat), 30g carb, 2g dietary fibre, 234 Cals (977kJ)

make it your way

DAIRY FREE Swap the milk for soy milk (contains soy) or another plant-based milk, and the chocolate for dairy-free chocolate.

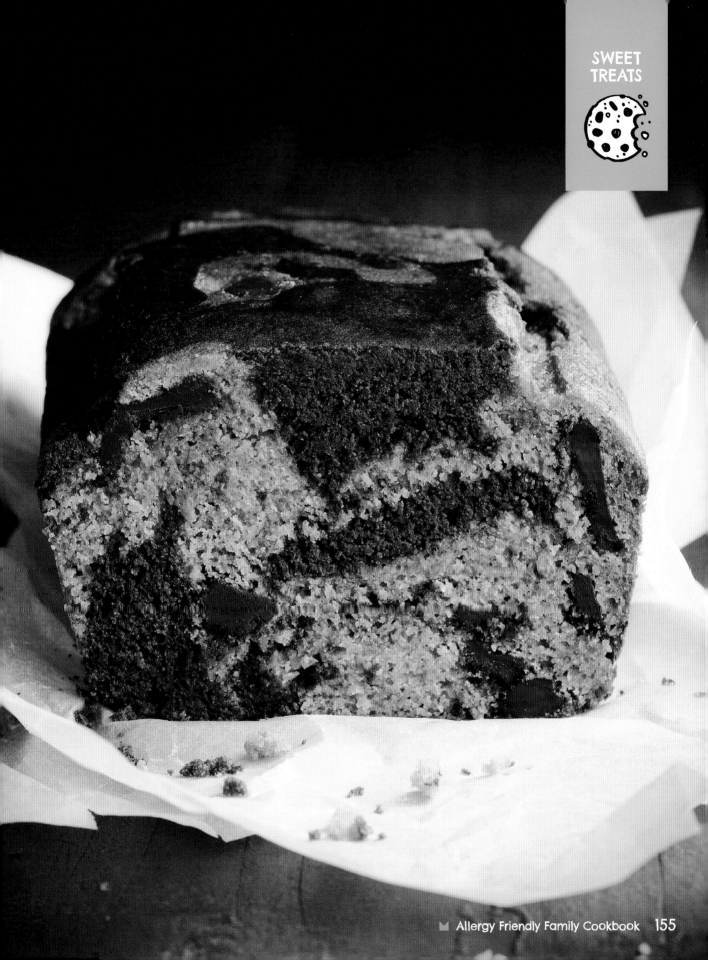

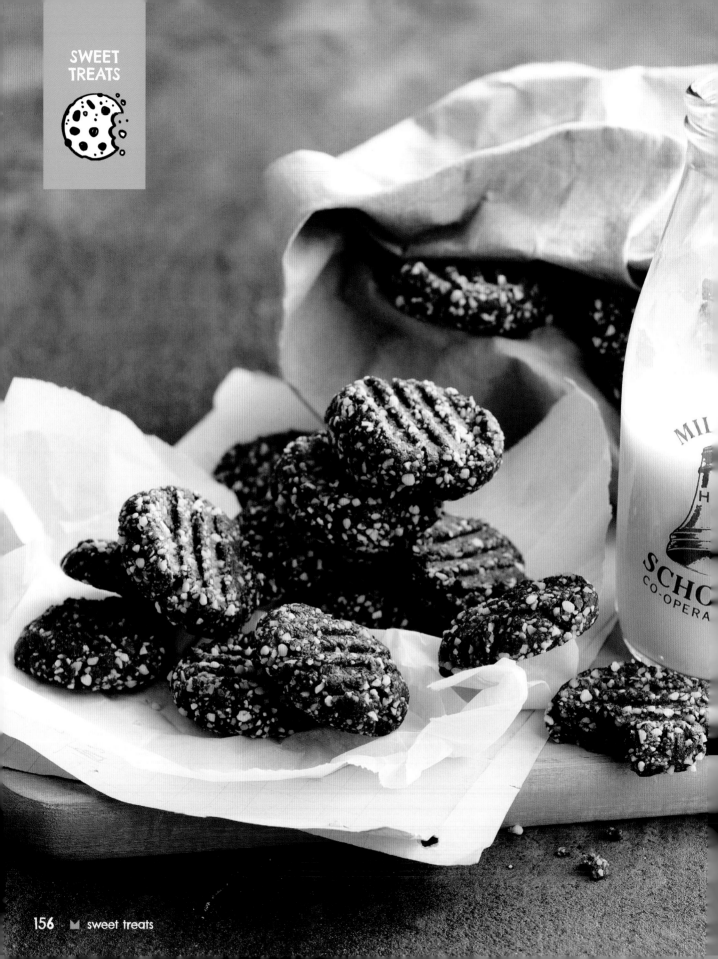

flourless choc-nut
BISCUITS

Skip the wheat, dairy and refined sugar, and indulge in these brilliant bikkies that are super easy to make and taste amazing.

makes 30   prep 20 mins (+ cooling)   cook 15 mins

ingredients

110g (¾ cup) roasted unsalted cashews
110g (¾ cup) macadamias
30g (¼ cup) sesame seeds
225g (1½ cups) fresh dates, pitted
1½ tbs raw cacao powder (or cocoa powder)

1　Preheat oven to 170°C/150°C fan forced. Line 2 baking trays with baking paper. Place all ingredients in a food processor and process for 1 minute or until nuts are finely chopped and the mixture is well combined and smooth.

2　Roll 2 tsp mixture into a ball. Place on the prepared tray. Repeat with the remaining mixture to make about 30 balls. Use a fork to flatten slightly. Bake for 10-12 minutes or until lightly coloured (biscuits will still be soft). Cool on trays for 5-10 minutes. Transfer to a wire rack to cool completely, before serving.

PER SERVE 1g protein, 5g fat (1g saturated fat), 6g carb, 1g dietary fibre, 78 Cals (323kJ)

make it your way

SESAME FREE Replace sesame seeds with pepitas or sunflower seed kernels. BOOST Pop ½ tsp cinnamon or ground cardamom into the food processor in step 1. MAKE AHEAD Freeze uncooked biscuits in an airtight container for up to 2 months. Thaw and bake, to serve.

granny's apple
CRUMBLE

Gluten-free almond meal combines with coconut and cinnamon in this warming retro apple dessert.

serves 6   prep 25 mins (+ cooling)   cook 40 mins

ingredients

6 Granny Smith apples, peeled, cored, cut into wedges
2 tbs fresh lemon juice
2 tbs caster sugar
1 tsp pure vanilla extract
Pure icing sugar, to dust
Gluten-free vanilla ice-cream, to serve

crumble

50g (⅓ cup) gluten-free plain flour
40g (⅓ cup) almond meal
35g (½ cup) shredded coconut
1 tsp ground cinnamon
60g (⅓ cup, firmly packed) brown sugar
60g unsalted butter, chopped
25g (¼ cup) flaked almonds

1 Preheat the oven to 180°C/160°C fan forced. Lightly grease a 1L (4 cup) round ovenproof dish.

2 Combine the apple, lemon juice, sugar, vanilla and 80ml (⅓ cup) water in a large saucepan. Cook, stirring occasionally, over medium heat for 10-15 minutes or until apples are tender. Transfer mixture to the prepared dish.

3 To make the crumble, combine the flour, almond meal, coconut, cinnamon and sugar in a bowl. Use fingertips to rub the butter into the flour mixture until the mixture resembles coarse breadcrumbs. Stir in the almonds.

4 Evenly sprinkle the crumble mixture over the apple mixture. Bake for 25 minutes or until golden. Cool for 5 minutes. Dust with icing sugar. Serve with ice-cream.

PER SERVE 5.1g protein, 22.7g fat (12.5g saturated fat), 48.4g carb, 5.2g dietary fibre, 425 Cals (1775kJ)

make it your way
DAIRY FREE Replace the butter with a chilled dairy-free butter blend, and serve with dairy-free ice-cream or coconut yoghurt.

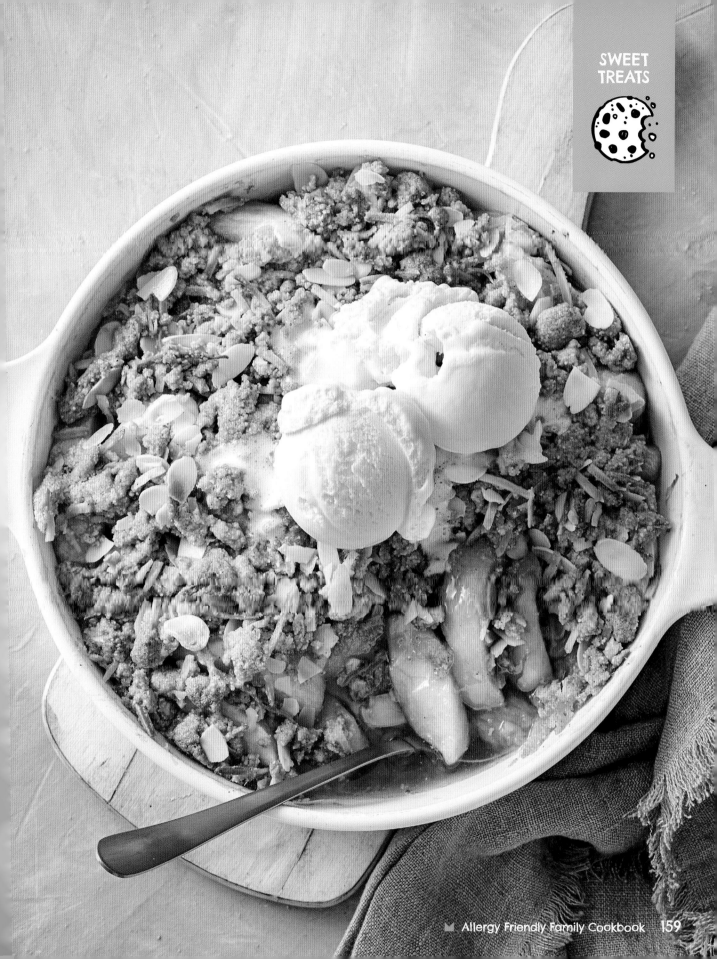

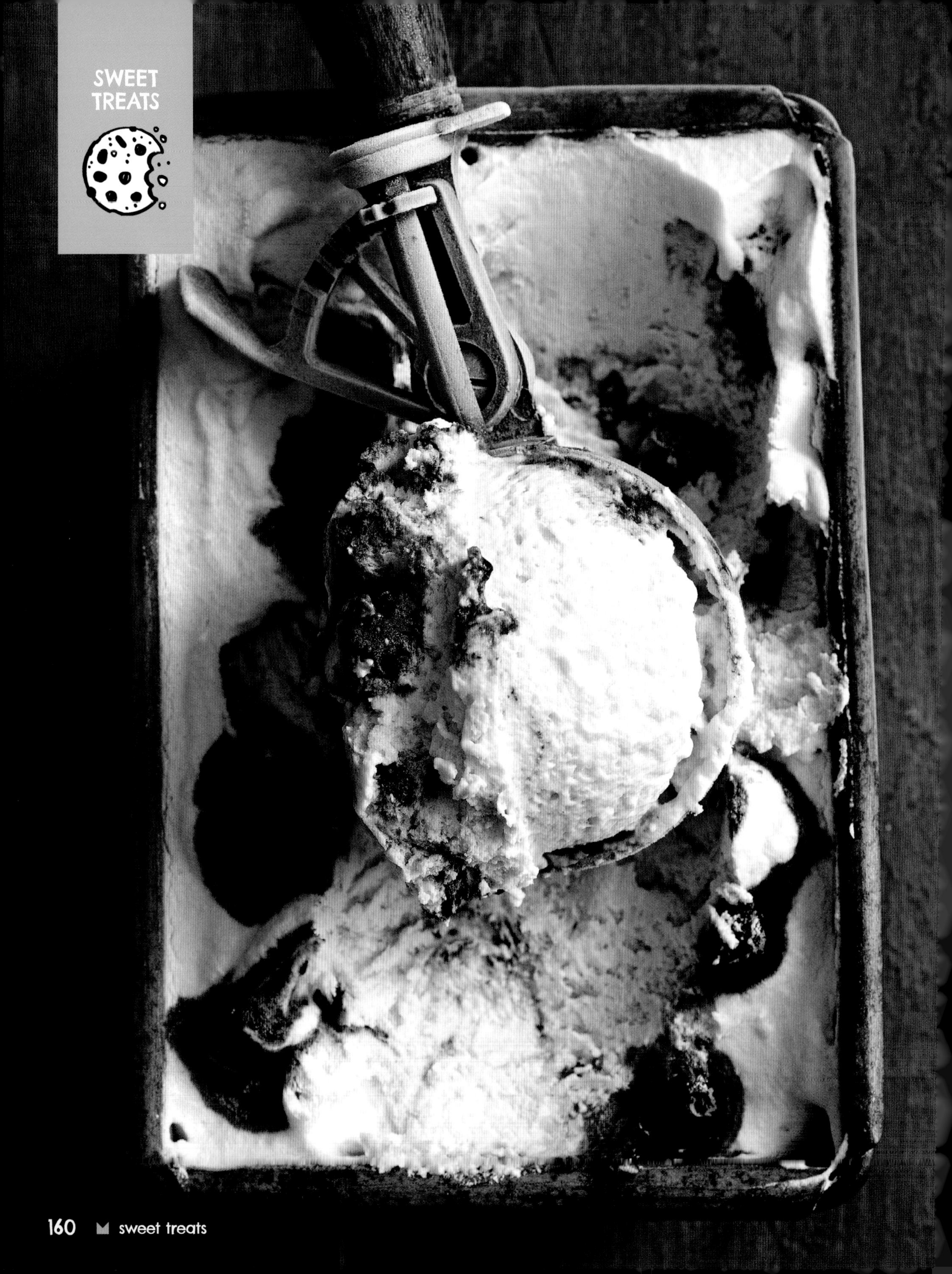

blueberry-swirl coconut
ICE-CREAM

A dairy-free ice-cream that's gluten free and deliciously creamy.
It needs a bit of freezer time, so start the recipe two days before serving.

makes 1L   prep 25 mins (+ 8 hours freezing & 4 hours or overnight chilling)   cook 15 mins

ingredients

125g fresh blueberries
2 tsp liquid glucose, plus
   extra 130g (⅓ cup)
40g (¼ cup) coconut sugar
1 tsp vanilla extract
2 x 270ml cans coconut milk,
   chilled for 4 hours or overnight
4 egg whites

1 Place berries, glucose, 2 tsp sugar and half the vanilla in a saucepan over low heat. Cook, stirring occasionally, for 6 minutes or until sugar dissolves. Transfer to a bowl. Cool for 30 minutes. Place in fridge.

2 Scoop solidified coconut milk from surface in cans into a glass bowl to measure 220ml (see make it your way). Whisk until thickened slightly.

3 Use electric beaters with a whisk attachment to whisk egg whites in a bowl until firm peaks form. Place extra glucose and remaining sugar and vanilla in a saucepan over low heat. Cook, stirring, for 2 minutes or until sugar is almost dissolved. Bring to a simmer. Simmer, without stirring, until 118°C on a sugar thermometer. With motor running slowly, add syrup to egg white, whisking until combined. Whisk for a further 4 minutes or until thickened. Cool for 2 minutes. Fold in whipped milk.

4 Pour half coconut mixture into a 1.4L loaf pan. Spoon two-thirds of syrup randomly over top. Use a butter knife to create swirls. Repeat with syrup and butter knife. Freeze for 8 hours or until firm. Serve.

PER SERVE 3.5g protein, 16.4g fat (14.5g saturated fat), 28.5g carb, 1.9g dietary fibre, 260 Cals (1087kJ)

make it your way

USE IT UP You can use the leftover coconut milk in many recipes in this book. Try the banoffee coconut puddings on page 177.

nice 'n' tangy
LEMON SLICE

These sweet gluten-free lemon bars are deliciously
zingy — perfect for an afternoon tea or anytime treat.

makes 16   prep 20 mins (+ cooling)   cook 40 mins

ingredients

100g (½ cup) caster sugar
75g (½ cup) gluten-free
    plain flour
55g (½ cup) almond meal
45g (½ cup) desiccated coconut
100g unsalted butter, melted
Pure icing sugar, sifted,
    to dust
Small lemon slices & whipped
    cream, to decorate (optional)

lemon filling

4 eggs
35g (¼ cup) gluten-free
    plain flour
215g (1 cup) caster sugar
1 lemon, rind finely grated
125ml (½ cup) fresh lemon juice

1 Preheat oven to 180°C/160°C fan forced. Line a 16 x 26cm (base size)
slice pan with baking paper, allowing the sides to overhang.

2 Combine the sugar, flour, almond meal and coconut in a bowl.
Add the butter and stir until well combined. Press mixture firmly
over the base of the prepared pan and smooth the surface. Bake for
15 minutes or until light golden.

3 To make the filling, whisk the eggs, flour and sugar in a bowl until
smooth. Whisk in the lemon rind and juice.

4 Carefully pour filling over the base. Bake for 20-25 minutes or until
filling is set. Cool completely in the pan before cutting into pieces
and dusting with icing sugar. Decorate with small lemon slices and
piped whipped cream, if desired.

PER SERVE 2.9g protein, 10g fat (5.4g saturated fat), 26.1g carb,
1.1g dietary fibre, 205 Cals (855kJ)

make
it your
way

DAIRY FREE Use a dairy-free spread and dairy-free cream to whip.
CHANGE IT UP Swap the lemon juice, rind and slices for orange.

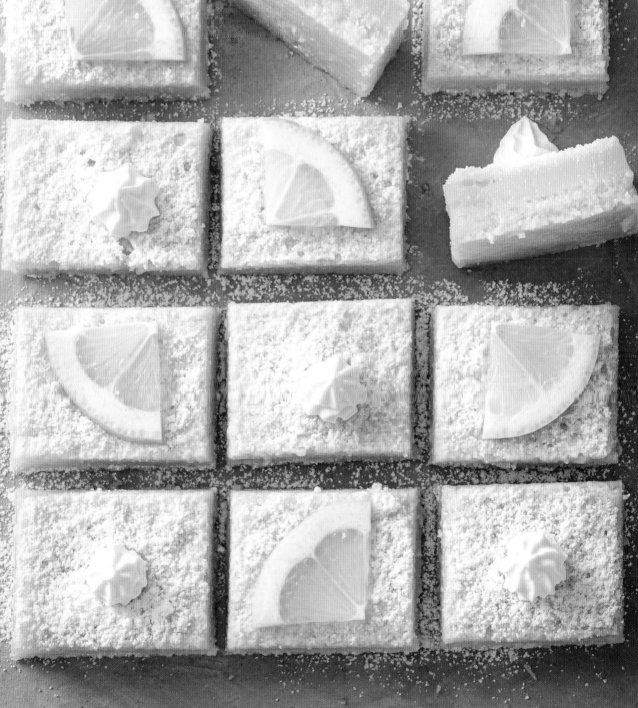

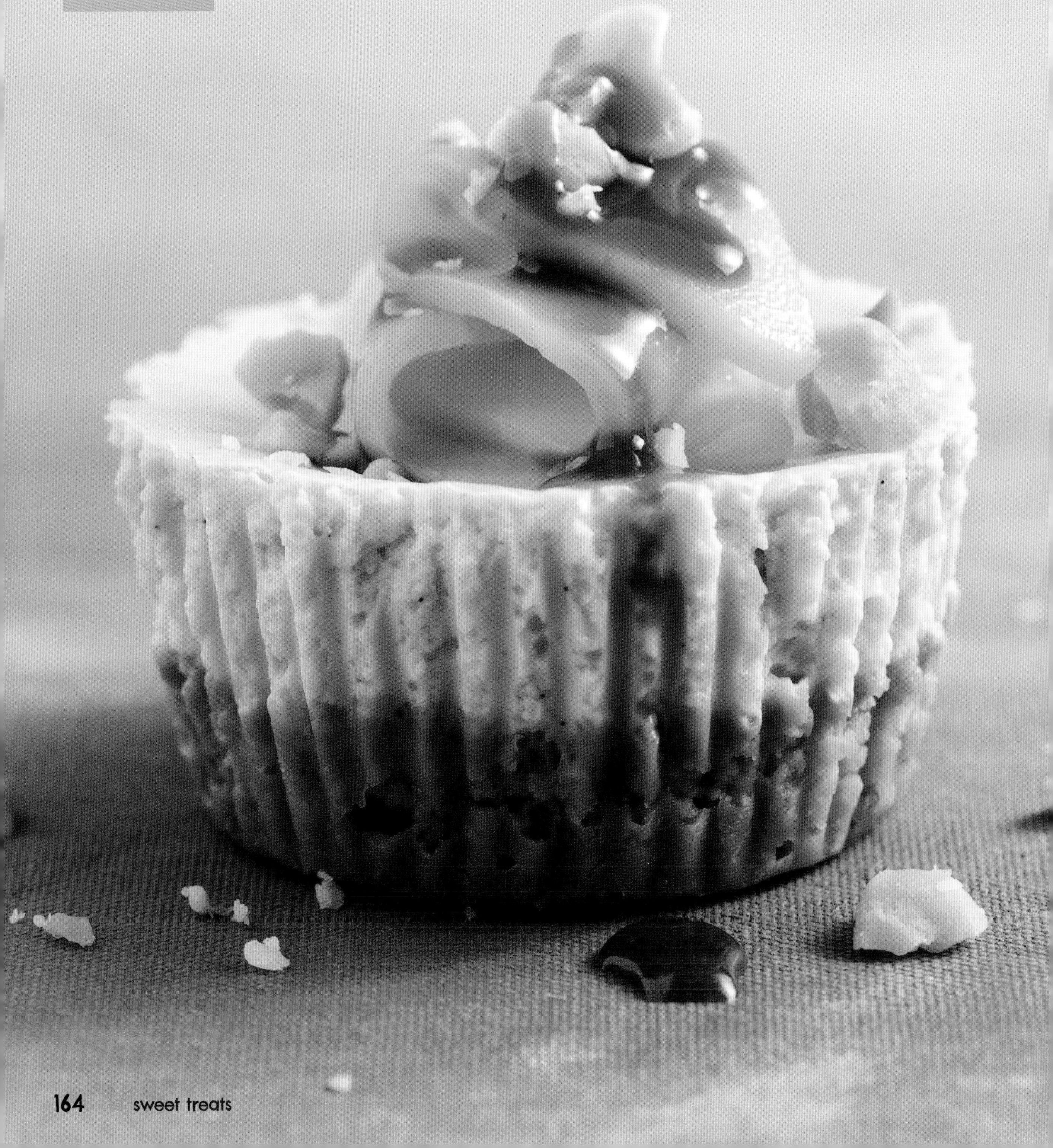

dairy-free caramel
CHEESECAKES

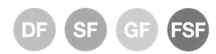

Anyone for dessert? No-one will guess these creamy caramel cheesecakes are both gluten and dairy free!

makes 12   prep 40 mins (+ cooling & 2 hours chilling)   cook 45 mins

ingredients

275g dairy-free, gluten-free arrowroot biscuits
70g cacao butter, melted
300g silken tofu, chopped into cubes
2 eggs
1 tsp vanilla bean paste
4 tbs coconut sugar
400ml can coconut cream
Pinch of salt flakes
1 mango, thinly sliced
Roasted macadamias, coarsely chopped, to serve

1 Preheat oven to 170°C/150°C fan forced. Line a 12-hole 80ml muffin pan with paper cases. Process biscuits in a food processor until fine crumbs form. Add butter and process to combine. Divide mixture among paper cases, pressing firmly into bases. Bake for 15 minutes or until golden. Cool in the pan.

2 Process tofu, eggs, vanilla, 1 tbs sugar and 300ml coconut cream in the food processor until smooth. Transfer to a jug. Evenly pour over cooled bases. Bake for 15-20 minutes or until filling is just set. Cool in the pan, then place in the fridge for 2 hours or until cold.

3 Combine remaining coconut sugar and 2 tbs water in a small saucepan. Heat over low heat until sugar melts. Increase heat to medium. Bring to the boil. Reduce heat to low. Simmer for 3-4 minutes or until deep caramel in colour. Add remaining coconut cream. Simmer for 5 minutes or until slightly reduced. Remove from the heat. Stir in the salt. Cool.

4 To serve, fold mango slices into curls and arrange on cheesecakes. Sprinkle with macadamia and drizzle with caramel sauce.

PER SERVE 7g protein, 9g fat (4g saturated fat), 24g carb, 2g dietary fibre, 215 Cals (898kJ)

make it your way

NUT FREE Swap the macadamias for finely chopped strawberries.
BOOST Serve with a large dollop of dairy-free thickened cream.

chocolate + avocado
MOUSSE TART

Indulge in this dairy-free dessert that uses avocado
and banana to create a wonderfully rich mousse filling.

serves 4   prep 30 mins (+ cooling & 2 hours chilling)   cook 20 mins

ingredients

2 tsp solid coconut oil,
   to grease, plus extra
   60g (¼ cup), melted
1 egg, lightly whisked
230g (2¼ cups) hazelnut meal
30g (¼ cup) Dutch-processed
   cocoa powder
1 tbs dark agave syrup
125g strawberries
125g fresh raspberries

avocado mousse

2 small ripe avocados, chopped
1 large over-ripe banana,
   chopped
60g (½ cup) Dutch-processed
   cocoa powder
1 tsp vanilla bean paste
185g (½ cup) dark agave syrup
2 egg whites

1 Preheat oven to 180°C/160°C fan forced. Place a baking tray in the oven. Grease a 2cm-deep, 22cm round (base size) loose-based fluted tart pan with coconut oil.

2 Combine the egg, hazelnut meal, cocoa, agave syrup and extra coconut oil in a bowl. Press firmly over base and side of prepared pan. Place pan on the hot tray. Bake for 20 minutes or until golden. Cool completely.

3 To make the avocado mousse, process the avocado, banana, cocoa, vanilla and agave syrup in a food processor until smooth and combined. Transfer to a large bowl.

4 Use an electric mixer to beat egg whites until soft peaks form. Fold, in 2 batches, into the avocado mixture. Spoon into pan and smooth the surface. Place in the fridge for 2 hours or until set. Decorate with berries. Serve immediately or keep in the fridge until serving.

PER SERVE 6.6g protein, 24.8g fat (7.9g saturated fat), 18.8g carb, 3.4g dietary fibre, 326 Cals (1366kJ)

make it your way

TRY Top with fresh blackberries and dust with gluten-free icing sugar.
BOOST Serve with a large dollop of cashew cream or coconut cream.

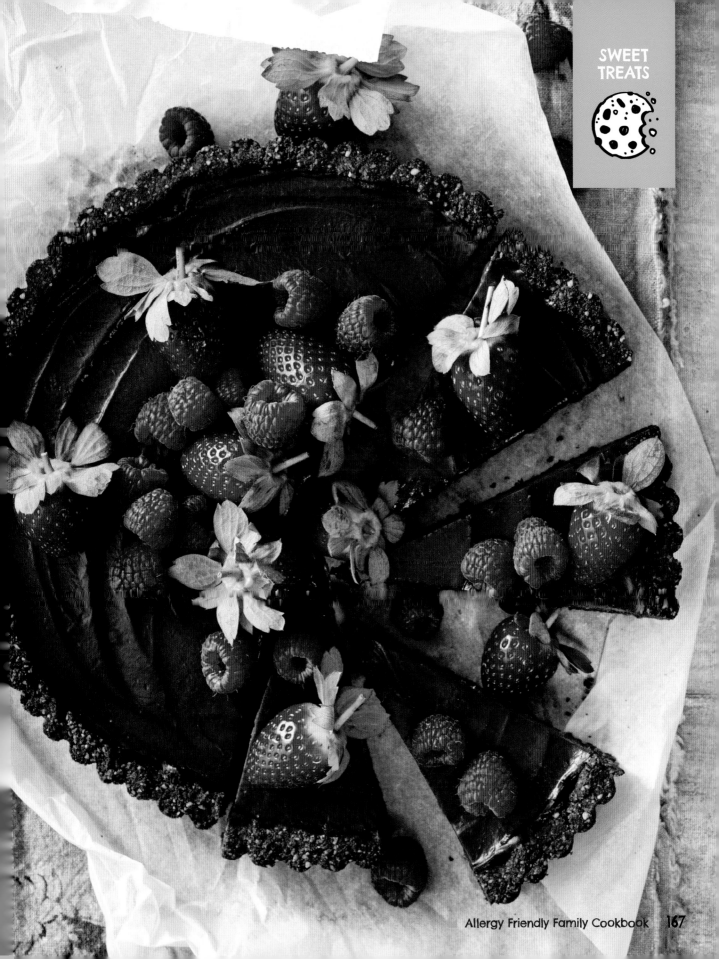

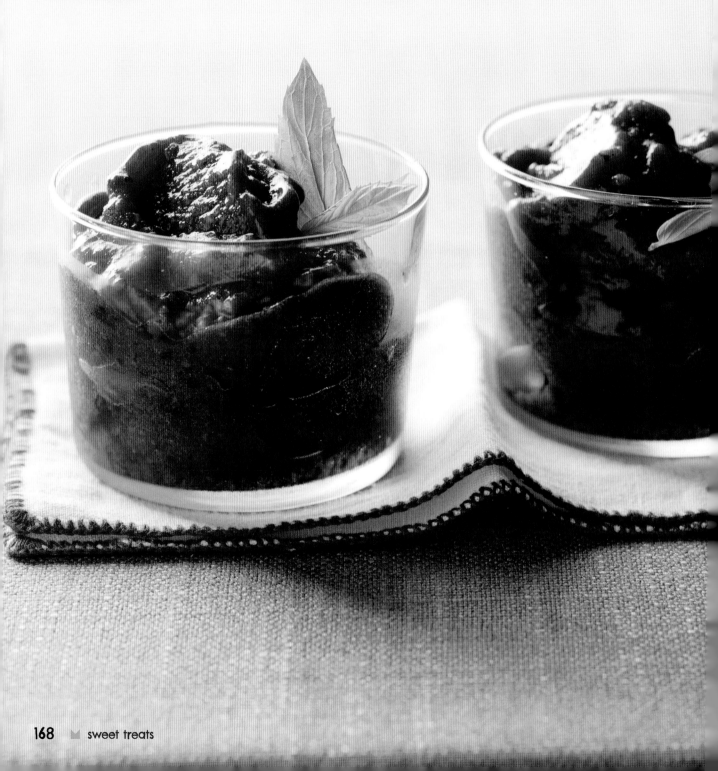

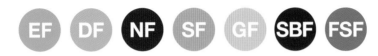

raspberry, mint + apple
SORBET

EF **DF** **NF** **SF** **GF** **SBF** **FSF**

Ready to serve in just 5 minutes, let this tangy sorbet be your dessert go-to on summer evenings and when entertaining.

makes 4   prep 5 mins

ingredients

500g pkt frozen raspberries
2 tbs fresh mint leaves, torn,
    plus extra leaves, to serve
375ml (1½ cups) chilled
    apple juice

1 Place the raspberries, mint leaves and 250ml (1 cup) apple juice in a food processor. Process, gradually adding remaining apple juice and scraping down side of processor occasionally, until smooth and well combined.

2 Working quickly, scoop mixture into serving glasses. Serve topped with extra mint leaves.

PER SERVE 0.0g protein, 0.7g fat (0.01g saturated fat), 17.0g carb, 7.0g dietary fibre, 100 Cals (100kJ)

make it your way

SEED FREE Not a fan of raspberry seeds? Push the blended mixture through a sieve. You will then need to freeze it for about 10 minutes so that it firms up again. SPIKE IT Replace the apple juice with orange juice and a dash of white rum to make a frozen daiquiri.

gluten- + dairy-free
DOUGHNUTS

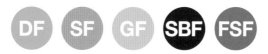

Everyone should get to enjoy warm, fluffy cinnamon doughnuts — and now they can with this easy baked recipe.

makes 6   prep 15 mins (+ cooling)   cook 15 mins

ingredients

130g (1 cup) gluten- and
   soy-free plain flour
½ tsp xanthan gum
1 tsp gluten-free baking powder
½ tsp salt
100g (½ cup) caster sugar
2 tsp ground cinnamon
1 egg, lightly whisked
1 tsp vanilla extract
125ml (½ cup) vegetable oil
80ml (⅓ cup) almond milk
1 tsp white vinegar

1 Preheat the oven to 220°C/200°C fan forced. Grease a six-hole doughnut pan.

2 Combine the flour, xanthan gum, baking powder, salt, half the sugar and half the cinnamon in a large bowl. Add the egg, vanilla, oil, almond milk and vinegar. Stir to combine. Spoon or pipe batter into prepared pan holes, keeping batter clear from doughnut holes and filling to about two-thirds full.

3 Bake for 10-12 minutes or until a skewer inserted into a doughnut comes out clean. Set aside for 5 minutes to cool slightly before transferring to a wire rack.

4 Combine the remaining sugar and cinnamon in a bowl. Place the doughnuts, one at a time, in the cinnamon sugar to coat. Serve warm or at room temperature.

PER SERVE 1.9g protein, 20.5g fat (2.3g saturated fat), 35g carb, 0.9g dietary fibre, 333 Cals (1393kJ)

make it your way

NUT FREE Instead of almond milk, choose a nut-free plant-based milk or cow's milk (contains dairy).

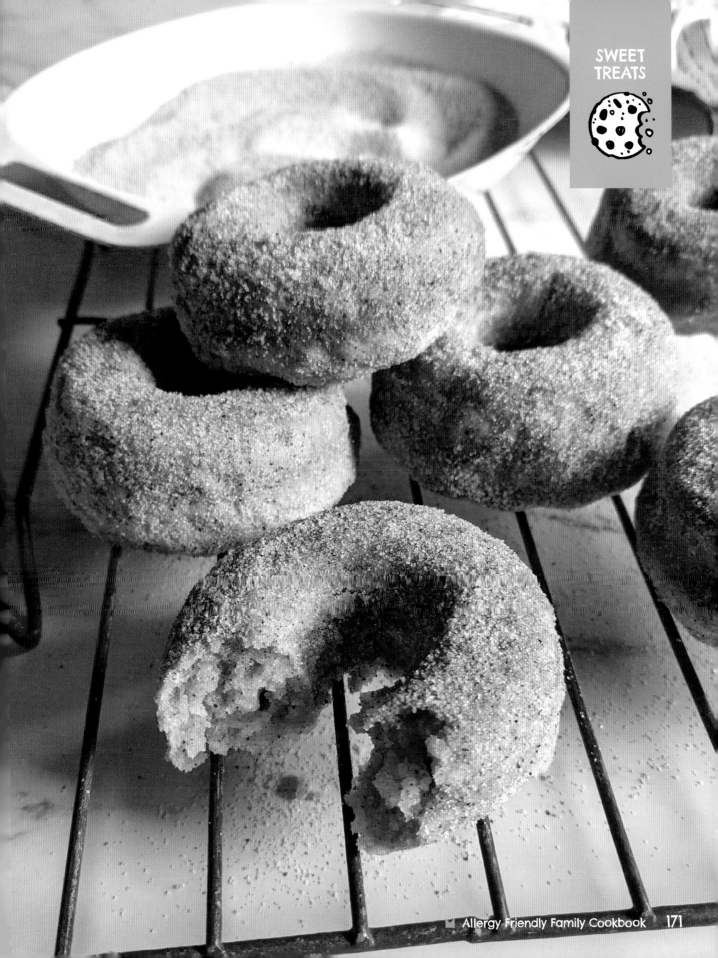

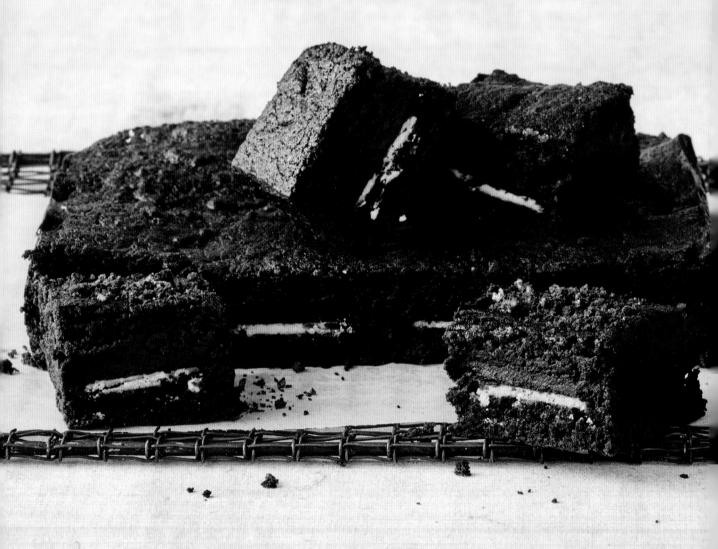

dairy-free oreo
BROWNIES

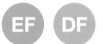

EF **DF** **NF** **SF** **FSF**

These gooey and fudgy chocolate brownies are stuffed with Oreo biscuits for the ultimate easy vegan treat.

makes 16   prep 25 mins   cook 40 mins

ingredients

2 tbs flaxseed meal

150g dairy-free chocolate, chopped

110g (½ cup) solid coconut oil

2 tsp vanilla extract

150g (1 cup) plain flour

155g (¾ cup, firmly packed) brown sugar

35g (⅓ cup) cocoa powder

¼ tsp bicarbonate of soda

16 Oreo biscuits

1 Preheat the oven to 160°C/140°C fan forced. Lightly grease a 20cm (base size) square cake pan. Line with baking paper, allowing the paper to overhang all sides.

2 Combine the flaxseed meal and 250ml (1 cup) water in a bowl. Set aside for 15 minutes to thicken. Meanwhile, combine the chocolate and coconut oil in a microwave-safe bowl. Microwave, stirring occasionally, for 2 minutes or until melted and smooth. Stir in vanilla.

3 Sift the flour, sugar, cocoa powder and bicarb into a large mixing bowl. Make a well in the centre. Add the chocolate mixture and flaxseed mixture to the well. Fold in until just combined. Spread half the mixture into the prepared pan.

4 Arrange the Oreos in a single layer over the top of the mixture in the pan, then spread remaining mixture over the top. Bake for 40 minutes. Cool completely in the pan. Use paper to lift out brownie slab. Use a sharp knife to cut into squares, to serve.

PER SERVE 2.6g protein, 12.5g fat (8.4g saturated fat), 32.8g carb, 1.3g dietary fibre, 240 cals (1005kJ)

make it your way

BOOST Leave brownie slab whole and decorate with hulled chopped strawberries. Serve with dairy-free thickened cream.

healthier tea-time
LEMON SLICE

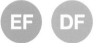

Imagine if we told you we'd made the classic lemon slice free of refined sugar, gluten and dairy? Imagine no more!

makes 12   prep 10 mins (+ cooling & chilling)   cook 15 mins

ingredients

165g (1⅓ cups) gluten- and
    soy-free plain flour
55g (½ cup) almond meal
20g (¼ cup) desiccated
    coconut, plus extra,
    toasted, to decorate
125ml (½ cup) light olive oil
125ml (½ cup) maple syrup
1 lemon, rind finely grated,
    plus extra lemon rind,
    shredded, to serve

coconut icing

400ml can coconut cream,
    chilled for 6 hours or overnight
2 tbs maple syrup

1 Preheat oven to 180°C/160°C fan forced. Grease the base and sides of a square 20cm (base size) baking pan. Line with baking paper, allowing the sides to overhang.

2 Whisk the flour, almond meal and coconut in a large bowl. Add the oil, maple syrup and lemon rind. Use a large metal spoon to stir until well combined. Evenly press mixture into the base of the prepared pan.

3 Bake base for 15 minutes or until lightly golden. Set pan aside for 30 minutes or until cooled completely.

4 To make coconut icing, scoop solid coconut cream (it will be a bit over half the can) into a bowl (save remaining coconut water for another use). Add maple syrup to the bowl. Use electric beaters or a stick blender to whip the cream mixture until thick and smooth. Pour over the prepared base. Place in the fridge for 30 minutes or until the icing is set. Sprinkle with the extra coconut and lemon rind. Keep in the fridge until ready to slice and serve.

PER SERVE 2.2g protein, 21.8g fat (9.5g saturated fat), 23.7g carb, 1g dietary fibre, 297 Cals (1244kJ)

make it your way

GIFT IT Turn this treat into a lovely gift for someone with allergies. Wrap a few bars in clear cellophane and secure with a pretty ribbon.

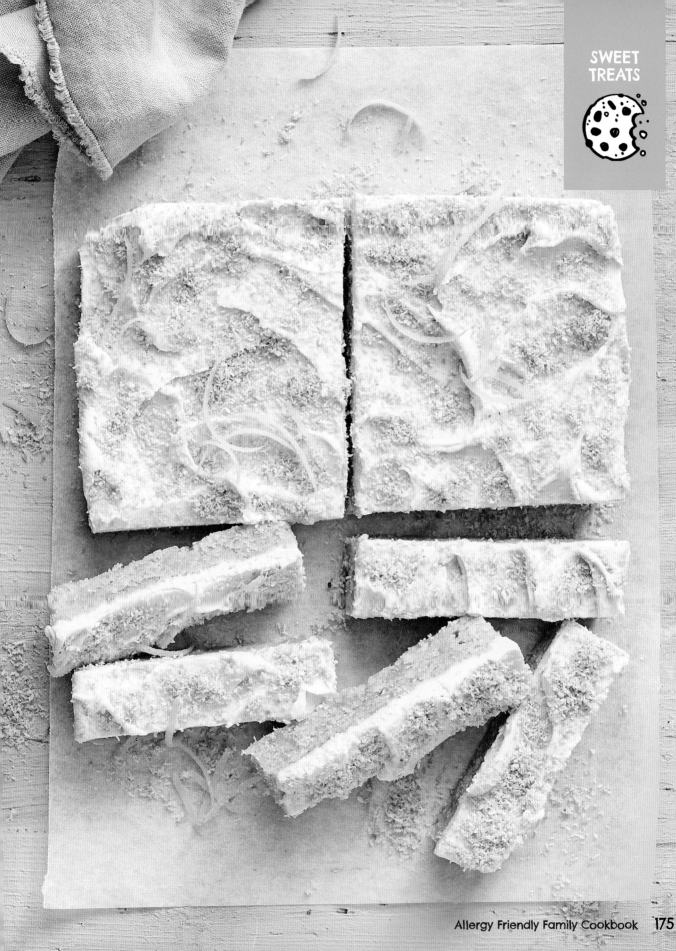

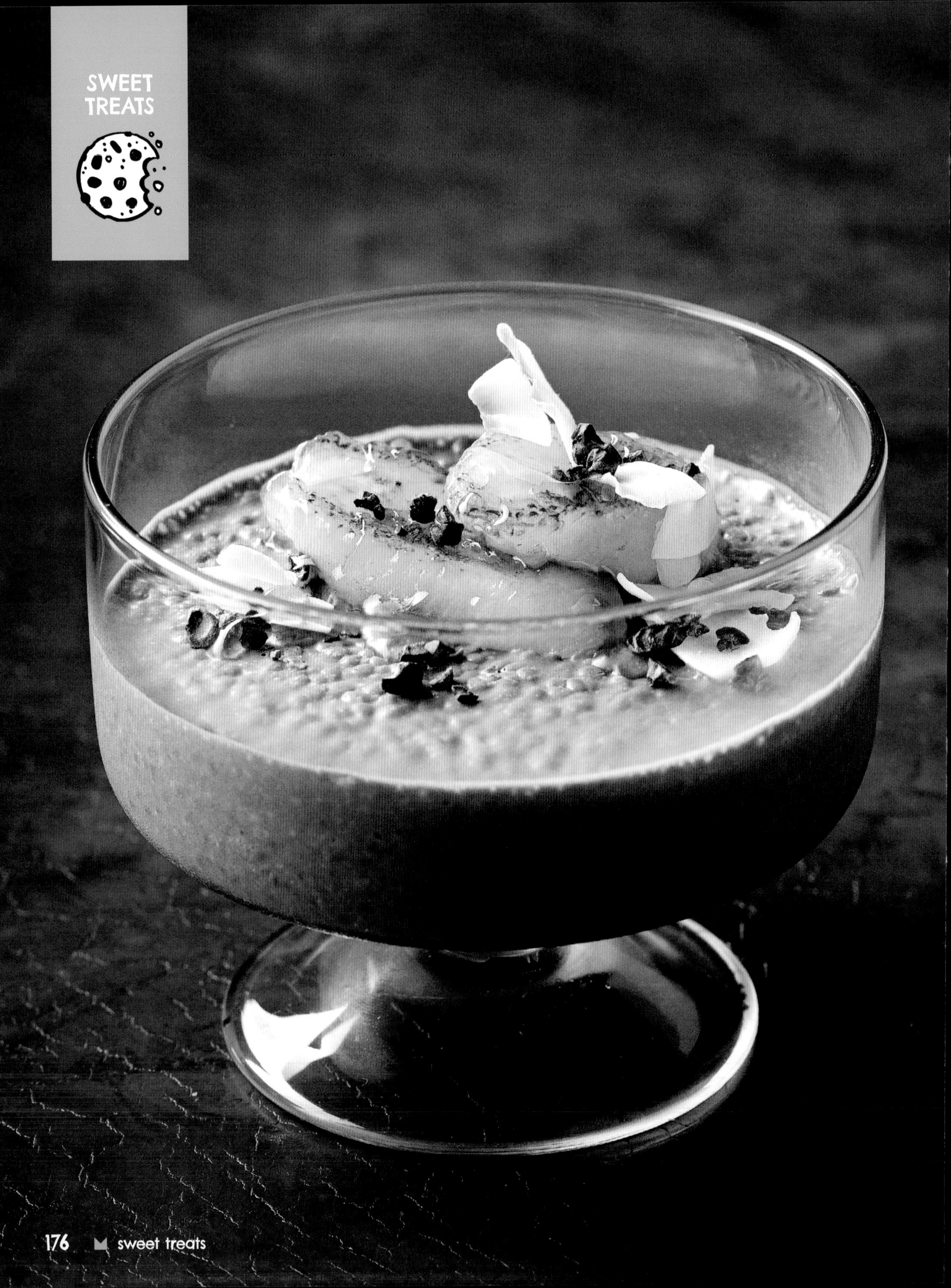

banoffee coconut
PUDDINGS

Make up a batch of these sweet coconut puds and have them on hand for a dairy-, gluten- and refined sugar-free dessert.

makes 4   prep 10 mins (+ 2 hours chilling)   cook 5 mins

ingredients

54g (¼ cup) black chia seeds
270ml can light coconut milk
2½ tbs raw cacao powder
60ml (¼ cup) rice malt syrup
1 tsp solid coconut oil
1 large banana, sliced
Pinch sea salt flakes
Roasted coconut chips and raw
   cacao nibs (optional), to serve

1 Place the chia seeds, coconut milk, cacao powder, 2 tbs water and 2 tbs rice malt syrup in a blender. Blend until almost smooth. Divide among four 125ml (½ cup) glasses. Place in fridge for 2 hours to chill.

2 Heat the oil in a non-stick frying pan over medium-high heat. Add the banana and cook for 30-60 seconds each side or until golden and caramelised. Remove from the heat. Sprinkle with sea salt. Drizzle with remaining rice malt syrup. Cool for 2 minutes.

3 Top the puddings with banana and drizzle with pan juices. Sprinkle with the coconut chips, and cacao nibs, if using. Serve.

PER SERVE 6.2g protein, 24.9g fat (17.4g saturated fat), 35.5g carb, 8.7g dietary fibre, 355 Cals (1485kJ)

MAKE IT A BREAKFAST Follow recipe to the end of Step 1. Top with sliced banana or berry compote and sprinkle with toasted chia seeds.

egg-free
MERINGUES

EF NF SF GF SBF FSF

These meringues are made using the liquid in a can of chickpeas (I know, right?), but are as sweet and crunchy as the real thing.

serves 6   prep 30 mins (+ cooling)   cook 2 hours

ingredients

400g can chickpeas, liquid
  only (reserve chickpeas for
  another use)
½ tsp cream of tartar
½ tsp white vinegar
150g (1 cup) pure icing sugar,
  sifted
1 tsp vanilla extract
300ml thickened cream,
  whipped

mixed berry syrup

55g (¼ cup) caster sugar
Pulp of 2 passionfruit
125g punnet fresh blueberries
250g punnet fresh strawberries,
  hulled, sliced

1 Preheat oven to 120°C/100°C fan forced. Use a pencil and 8cm round cutter to mark 6 circles, 4cm apart, on each of 2 sheets of baking paper. Line 2 large baking trays with the baking paper, marked-side down.

2 Beat 160ml (⅔ cup) chickpea liquid in an electric mixer for 5 minutes or until soft peaks form. Beat in cream of tartar and vinegar. Beat in icing sugar, 1 tbs at a time, until stiff glossy peaks form. Beat in vanilla. Fill a piping bag fitted with a 1cm fluted nozzle with meringue. Fill circles on prepared trays with meringue in a circular motion. Add a second layer. Bake for 2 hours or until just firm to touch. Turn off oven. Cool for 30 minutes in oven with door closed. Cool completely with door ajar.

3 Meanwhile, to make the syrup, place sugar, passionfruit and 125ml (½ cup) water in a saucepan over medium-high heat. Cook, stirring, for 2 minutes. Bring to the boil. Reduce heat to low. Simmer for 5 minutes or until thickened slightly. Add berries. Simmer for 1 minute. Let cool.

4 Spread 6 nests with cream. Top with half the berry syrup and the remaining nests. Top with remaining cream and berry syrup. Serve.

PER SERVE 2.1g protein, 18.7g fat (11.9g saturated fat), 37.7g carb, 2.1g dietary fibre, 324 Cals (1355kJ)

make
it your
way

DAIRY FREE Swap the cream for dairy-free cream or coconut yoghurt.
SEED FREE Strain the passionfruit pulp if you don't like the seeds.

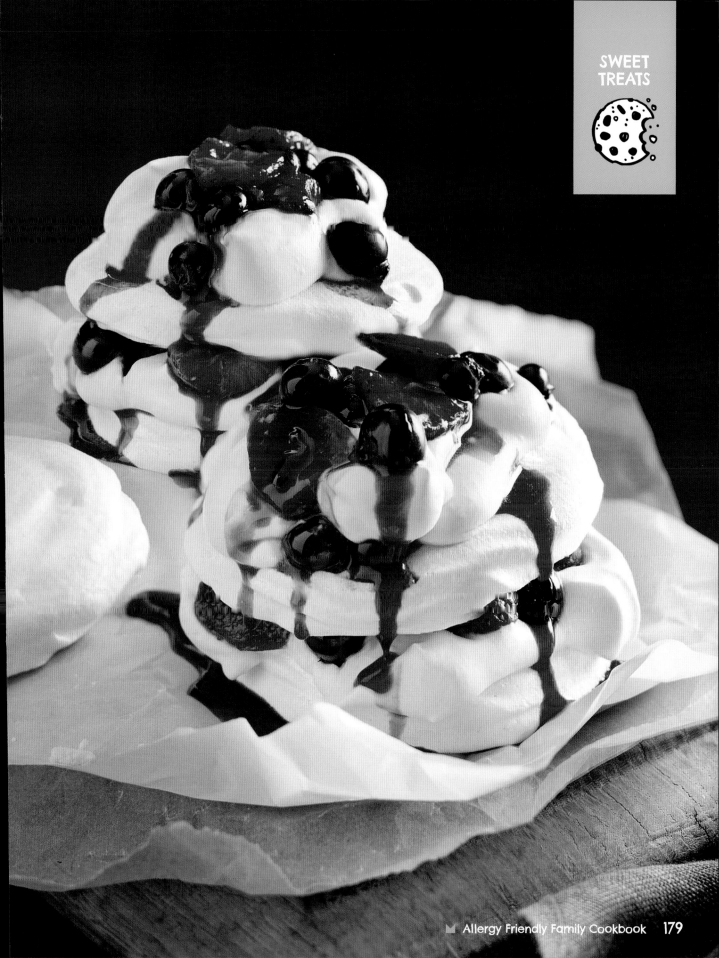

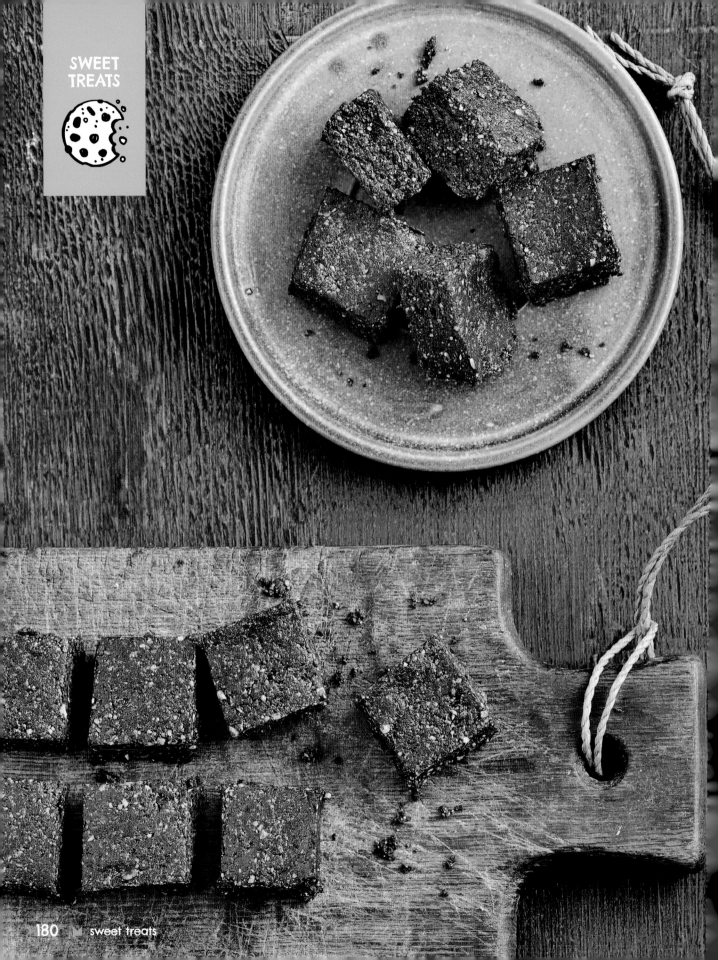

choc-hazelnut
FUDGE SLICE

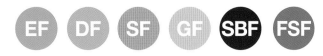

(EF) (DF) (SF) (GF) (SBF) (FSF)

No dairy, no gluten and just five ingredients to chocolate nutty goodness and an anytime treat.

makes 24   prep 15 mins (+ cooling & overnight chilling)   cook 5 mins

ingredients

120g pkt skinless hazelnuts
290g (1½ cups) medjool dates, pitted, halved
130g (½ cup) gluten-free almond spread
35g (⅓ cup) cocoa powder
2 tsp vanilla extract

1 Grease a 6cm-deep, 9 x 19cm (base size) loaf pan. Line with baking paper, extending paper 2cm above edges on all sides.

2 Place the hazelnuts in a large frying pan over medium heat. Cook, stirring, for 3-4 minutes or until golden and toasted. Transfer to a bowl. Cool completely.

3 Place the dates, almond spread, cooled hazelnuts, cocoa and vanilla in a food processor. Process until mixture comes together. Evenly press mixture over the base of the prepared pan. Cover. Place in the fridge overnight.

4 Use the baking paper to lift the fudge onto a board. Cut the slab into 24 small squares, to serve.

PER SERVE 2.3g protein, 7g fat (0.7g saturated fat), 7.9g carb, 1.6g dietary fibre, 102 Cals (425kJ)

make it your way

SWAP You can substitute the hazelnuts for peanuts, pecans, pistachios or almonds, whichever you prefer.

coconut
ETON MESS

Keep a can of coconut cream on stand-by in the fridge to whip up this quick and easy 4-ingredient dessert.

makes 2   prep 10 mins

ingredients

400g can coconut cream, chilled
   for 4 hours or overnight
1 mango, sliced
½ cup frozen raspberries,
   thawed
2 tbs sliced natural almonds,
   toasted

1 Turn can upside down. Open can and gently pour away coconut milk into a container (see make it your way). Spoon the solid coconut cream into the bowl of an electric mixer fitted with a whisk attachment. Beat for 1-2 minutes or until soft peaks form.

2 Divide one-third of the mango between 2 serving glasses. Top with half the whipped coconut cream. Top with raspberries and one-third of the mango. Dollop with remaining cream. Top with remaining mango and almonds, to serve.

PER SERVE 6.7g protein, 51.1g fat (42.6g saturated fat), 33g carb, 8.9g dietary fibre, 579 Cals (2424kJ)

make it your way

NUT FREE Omit nuts or swap for banana chips. USE IT UP Freeze the leftover coconut milk in ice-cube trays to use in smoothies.

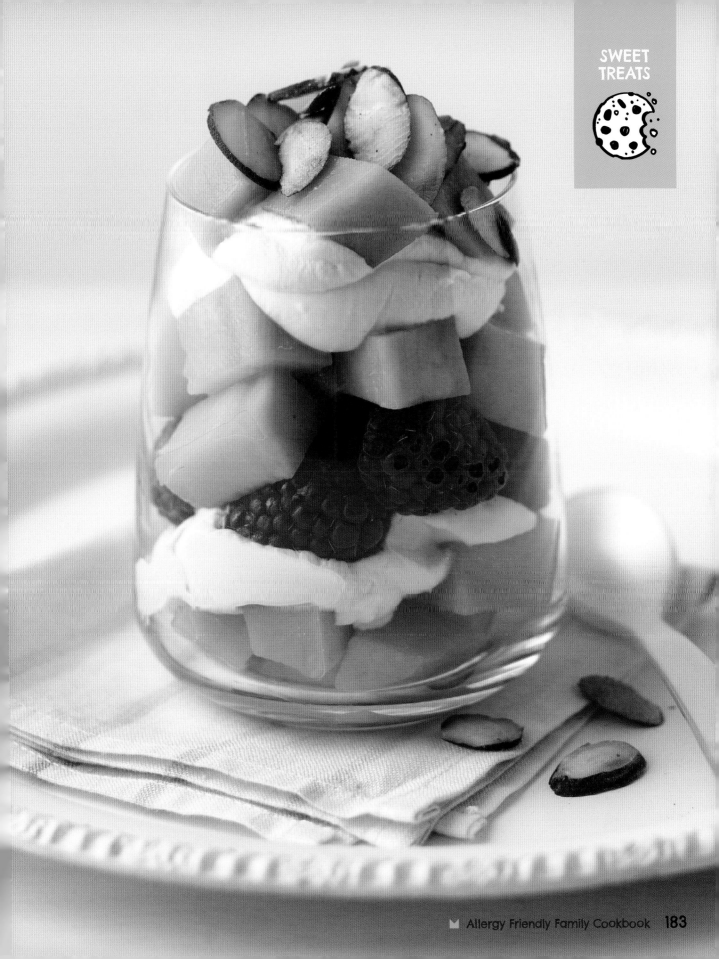

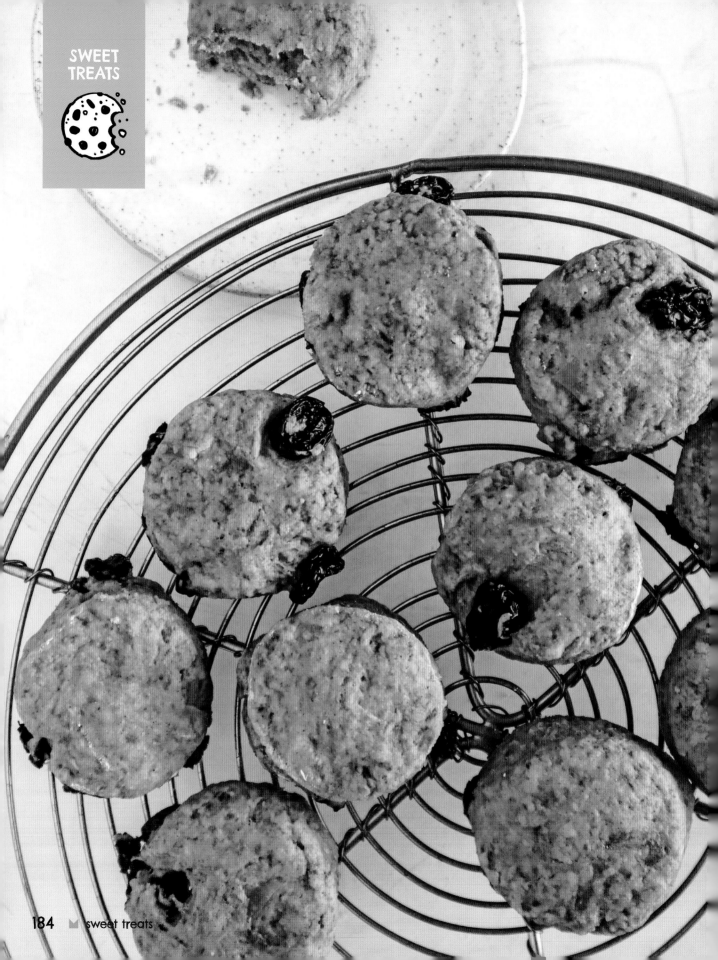

community recipe

mbatata

COOKIES

 EF DF NF SF SBF FSF

"Pronounced MM-ba-TA-ta, these yuMMy cookies from Malawi in Africa are soft and cakey. They're made with sweet potato, so they're a healthy yet still sweet alternative to regular cookies." *~ Tegan Laird*

makes 14   prep 15 mins (+ cooling)   cook 15 mins

ingredients

130g (½ cup) mashed sweet potato
2 tbs Nuttelex, melted
150g (1 cup) plain flour, plus extra, to dust
2 tsp baking powder
1 tsp ground cinnamon
45g (¼ cup) lightly packed brown sugar
¼ tsp salt
50g (¼ cup) raisins

1 Preheat the oven to 190°C/170°C fan forced. Line a large baking tray with baking paper.

2 Combine the sweet potato and Nuttelex in a large bowl. Sift the flour, baking powder and cinnamon into the bowl. Add the sugar and salt. Use a wooden spoon to mix and form a soft dough. Add the raisins and mix until combined.

3 Use clean hands to bring dough together. Turn onto on a lightly floured surface and gently knead, adding a little water if needed, until smooth. Use a rolling pin to roll out dough until 1.5cm thick. Use a 5cm round cookie cutter to cut out 14 rounds, gently re-rolling remaining dough, as needed.

4 Arrange dough rounds on prepared tray. Bake for 12-15 minutes or until firm but slightly springy to the touch. Cool on tray for 10 minutes, before transferring to a wire rack to cool completely. Serve.

PER SERVE 1.4g protein, 2.6g fat (0.6g saturated fat), 15g carb, 0.7g dietary fibre, 89 Cals (374kJ)

 make it your way

GLUTEN FREE Substitute the plain flour for gluten-free flour.
EAT FRESH These cookies are best eaten the day they are baked.

bonnie's
OAT SLICE

 EF NF SF SBF FSF

"We love this easy, delicious slice. The recipe was one of my first baking attempts after it was confirmed that Bonnie, my daughter, was allergic to eggs (since outgrown), peanuts and sesame. That was eight years ago. We've been baking this slice ever since." ~ *Claire Voss*

makes 18   prep 10 mins (+ cooling)   cook 20 mins

ingredients

90g (1 cup) gluten-free rolled oats (not quick oats)
150g (1 cup) plain flour
160g (1 cup) lightly packed brown sugar
45g (½ cup) desiccated coconut
125g unsalted butter
60ml (¼ cup) golden syrup
¼ tsp bicarbonate of soda

1 Preheat the oven to 160°C/140°C fan forced. Grease a 20 x 30cm (base size) slice pan. Line with baking paper, extending the paper over the 2 long sides.

2 Place the oats, flour, sugar and coconut in a large bowl. Stir to combine. Make a well in the centre.

3 Place the butter and golden syrup in a saucepan over low heat. Cook, stirring, until the butter melts and the mixture is smooth. Remove from the heat and stir in the bicarb – it will bubble up!

4 Pour the butter mixture into the well in the dry ingredients and stir to combine. Press mixture into the prepared pan. Smooth the surface.

5 Bake for 20 minutes or until slice is set and golden brown. Cool in the pan before lifting onto a board. Cut into 18 pieces, to serve.

PER SERVE 1.7g protein, 7.9g fat (5.3g saturated fat), 21g carb, 1g dietary fibre, 161 Cals (673kJ)

make it your way

GLUTEN FREE Use gluten-free plain flour.
DAIRY FREE Use any dairy-free butter in place of regular butter.

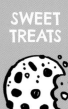

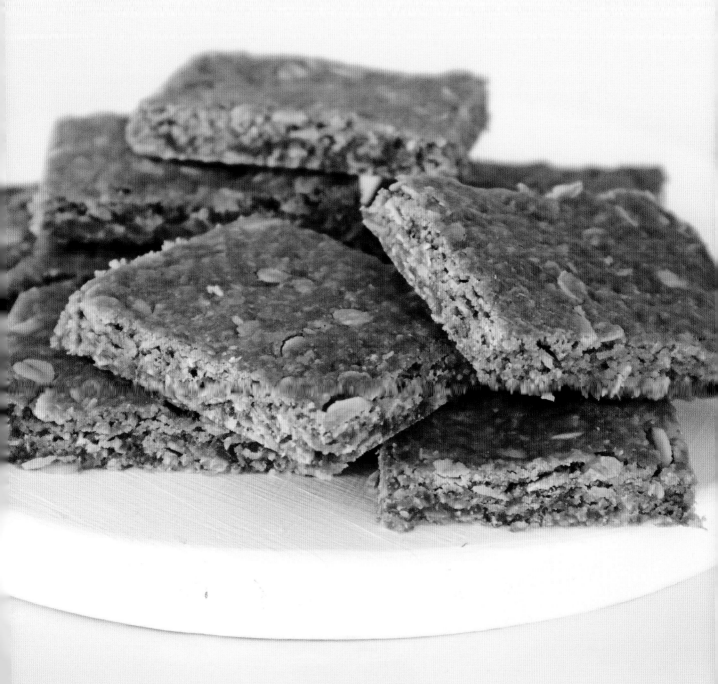

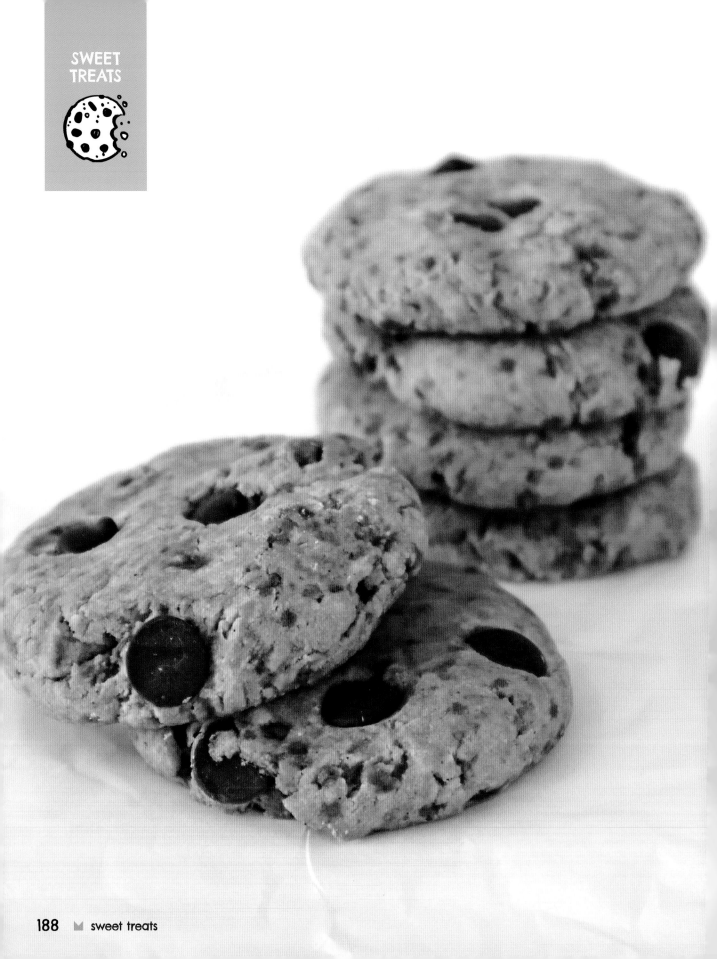

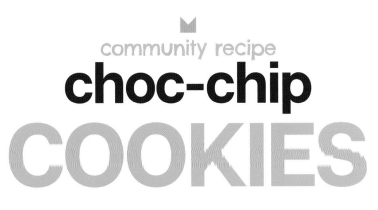

community recipe
choc-chip
COOKIES

EF **DF** **NF** **SF** **GF** **FSF**

"Choc-chip cookies are every child's favourite, and now they can still enjoy them even when allergies get in the way. These are wonderfully crunchy – be sure to keep the cookie jar full!" ~ *Karen Chetner*

makes 12   prep 15 mins (+ cooling)   cook 15 mins

ingredients

110g (½ cup) rapadura or
   raw sugar
80ml (⅓ cup) solid coconut
   oil, melted
1 large ripe banana, mashed
1 tsp vanilla extract
160g (1 cup) buckwheat flour
110g (¾ cup) quinoa flour
½ tsp bicarbonate of soda
¼ tsp sea salt flakes
45g (¼ cup) plant-based
   chocolate chips

1. Preheat the oven to 170°C/150°C fan forced. Line a large baking tray with baking paper. Use electric beaters to beat the sugar and coconut oil in a bowl until almost combined. Beat in the banana and vanilla until combined.

2. Add the flours, bicarb and salt to the bowl. Beat on low speed until combined. Stir in the chocolate chips.

3. Roll cookie dough into golf ball-sized balls. Place onto the prepared tray and flatten to about 1cm thick.

4. Bake cookies for 15 minutes or until golden underneath. Cool on the tray for 5 minutes. Transfer to a wire rack to cool completely. Serve.

PER SERVE 3.2g protein, 8.2g fat (6.4g saturated fat), 26.5g carb,
2.5g dietary fibre, 195 Cals (816kJ)

make it your way

SOY FREE Substitute the chocolate chips for soy-free chocolate chips.
TRY Swap chocolate for Smarties, which are dairy-, nut- and egg-free.

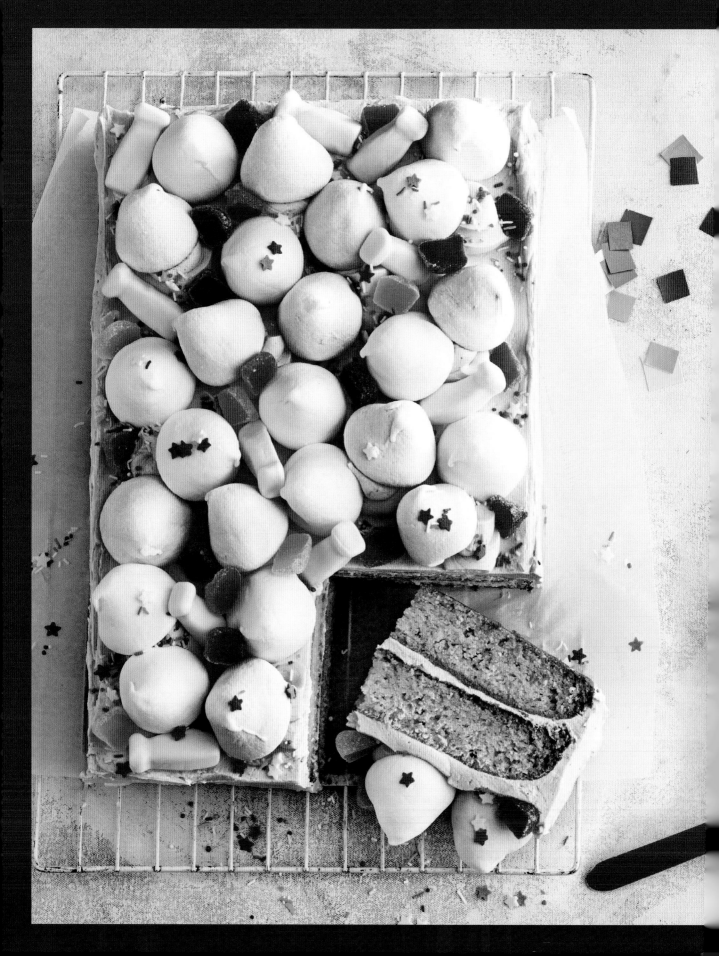

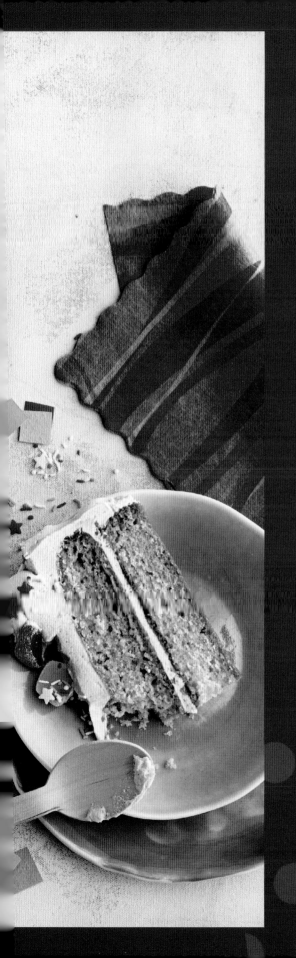

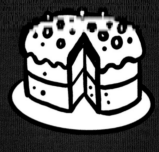

cakes

Whether it's for a birthday,
morning tea or 'just because',
we've got you covered.

strawberry-dusted LAYER CAKE

This heavenly strawberry cake number is worth
a celebration in itself. Go on, make an occasion of it.

serves 12   **prep** 45 mins (+ cooling & 20 mins chilling)   **cook** 50 mins

ingredients

420g (3 cups) buckwheat flour
1½ tbs gluten-free baking powder
200g (2 cups) almond meal
315g (1½ cups) caster sugar
4 eggs, lightly whisked
250ml (1 cup) sunflower oil
375ml (1½ cups) unsweetened
   almond milk
2 tsp vanilla bean paste
85g (¼ cup) strawberry jam
10g pkt freeze-dried strawberries,
   one-third crushed
Edible rose petals, to serve
   (optional)

pink frosting
250g Nuttelex spread
1 tsp vanilla bean paste
450g (3 cups) pure icing sugar
Pink gel food colouring, to tint

1 Preheat oven to 180°C/160°C fan forced. Grease two 6cm-deep, 20cm (base size) round cake pans. Line with 2 layers of baking paper. Sift half the flour, baking powder, almond meal and sugar into a bowl. Make a well. Stir half the whisked egg, oil, milk and vanilla into the well. Pour into prepared pans. Bake for 20-25 minutes or until a skewer inserted into centre of cakes comes out clean. Cool in pans for 10 minutes. Turn, top-side up, onto a wire rack to cool. Repeat to make 2 more cakes.

2 To make the frosting, use an electric mixer to beat the Nuttelex, vanilla and icing sugar until pale and fluffy. Use food colouring to tint pale pink.

3 Place 1 cake on a serving plate. Spread top with 1 tbs jam. Spread with ½ cup frosting. Top with a second cake. Continue layering with remaining jam, frosting and cakes. Use a palette knife to spread top and side of cake with remaining frosting. Scrape off some frosting to create a slightly 'naked' effect. Place in fridge for 20 minutes.

4 Top cake with whole freeze-dried strawberries. Decorate top and base with crushed strawberries and rose petals, if using. Serve.

PER SERVE 12.1g protein, 45.6g fat (5.3g saturated fat), 87g carb, 4.2g dietary fibre, 799 Cals (3343kJ)

GO FRESH Instead of using freeze-dried strawberries, you can decorate using fresh strawberries.

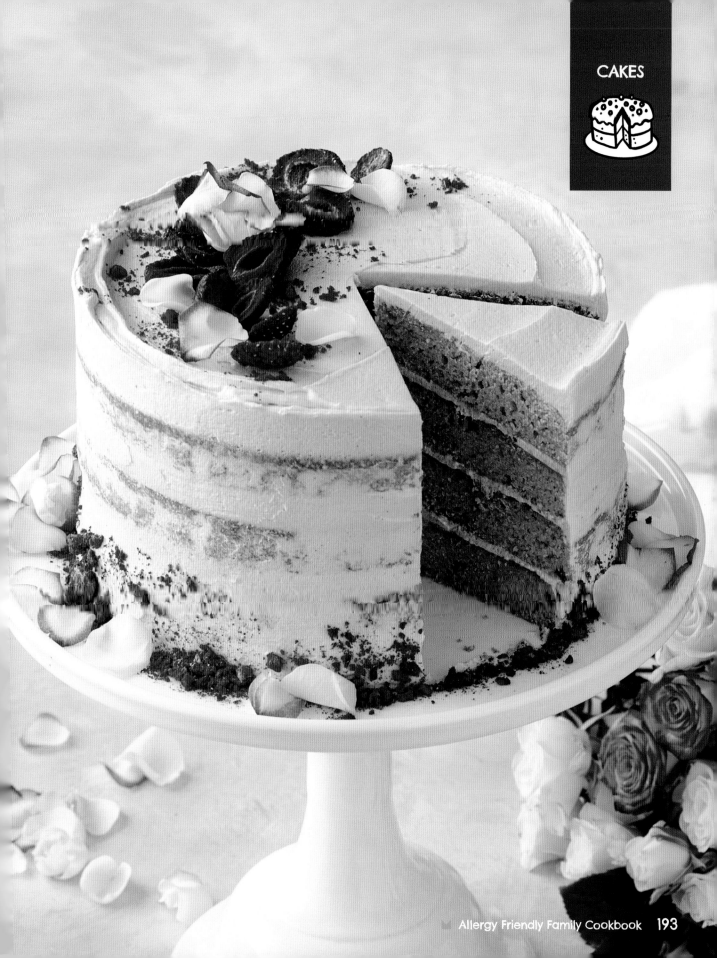

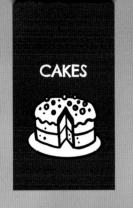

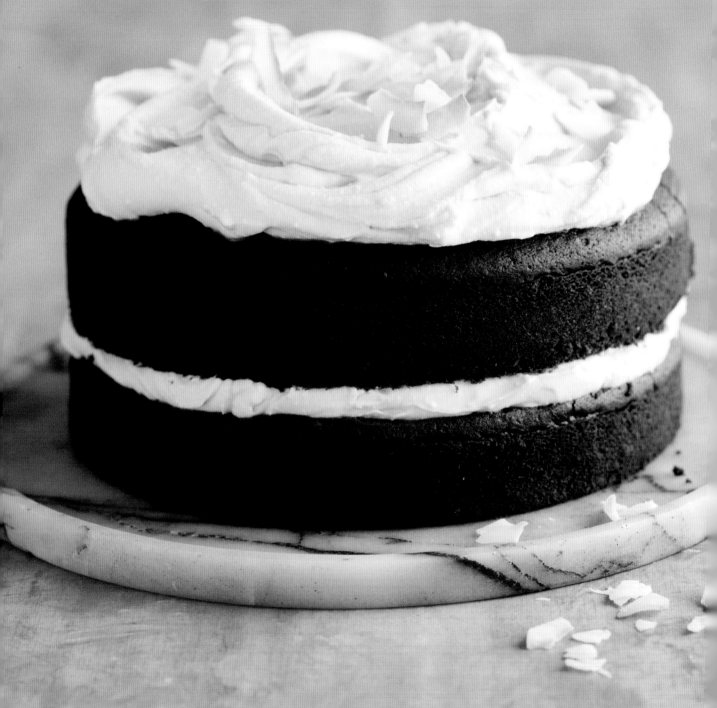

vegan choc-coconut CAKE

This delicious vegan cake is incredibly moist and has a light coconut frosting that will melt in your mouth.

serves 8   **prep** 30 mins (+ cooling)   **cook** 25 mins

ingredients

225g (1½ cups) plain flour
225g (1½ cups) self-raising flour
300g (1½ cups, firmly packed) brown sugar
50g (½ cup) cocoa powder
2 tsp bicarbonate of soda
Large pinch of salt
180ml (¾ cup) solid coconut oil, melted and cooled
60ml (¼ cup) black coffee, cooled
1½ tbs white wine vinegar
2 tsp vanilla bean paste

coconut frosting
2 x 400g cans coconut cream, chilled for 24 hours
45g (¼ cup) pure icing sugar
1 tsp vanilla bean paste
Coconut flakes, toasted, to decorate

1 Preheat oven to 180°C/160°C fan forced. Invert base, then line bases and sides of two 20cm (base size) springform pans.

2 Sift the flours, sugar, cocoa, bicarb and salt into a large bowl. Make a well in the centre. Add oil, coffee, vinegar, vanilla and 430ml (1¾ cups) water to the well. Use a large metal spoon to stir until combined.

3 Divide mixture evenly between prepared pans. Bake for 25 minutes or until cakes are springy to a gentle touch. Cool in pans for 10 minutes. Release cakes and transfer to a wire rack to cool completely.

4 Scoop thick coconut cream from the top of each can (reserve remaining coconut water for another use) and place in a bowl. Add icing sugar and vanilla. Use electric beaters to beat until thickened.

5 Place 1 cake on a serving plate and spread with half the frosting. Top with remaining cake and spread with the remaining frosting. Sprinkle top of cake with coconut. Keep in the fridge until ready to serve.

PER SERVE 8.9g protein, 43g fat (38.3g saturated fat), 87.8g carb, 4.7g dietary fibre, 772 Cals (3226kJ)

GO SMALLER Halve the ingredients and cook the cake in the one pan.
BOOST Decorate with fresh berries or grated vegan chocolate.

frozen tropical
DESSERT CAKE

EF **DF** **NF** **SF** **GF** **SBF** **FSF**

Looking for an easy dairy-free dessert? Try our frozen triple-layer cake made with sorbet and coconut-based ice-cream for a dreamy summer tropical escape.

serves 12   **prep** 15 mins (+ 10 mins standing & 3 hours freezing)

ingredients

1L mango sorbet
1L plant-based (coconut) vanilla 'ice-cream'
1L raspberry sorbet
Sliced fresh mango, fresh raspberries, fresh passionfruit pulp and shaved coconut, to serve

1 Line the base and side of a 23cm springform pan with baking paper. Remove mango sorbet from the freezer and set aside for 10 minutes or until softened slightly. Spoon the sorbet into the prepared pan, pressing down to form an even layer. Smooth the surface. Place in the freezer for 20 minutes or until firm.

2 Repeat with the coconut 'ice-cream' and raspberry sorbet, freezing each layer for 20 minutes or until firm. Cover the surface with plastic wrap and freeze all three layers for a further 2 hours or until firm.

3 Just before serving, release the side of the pan and transfer the cake to a serving plate. Top with the mango, raspberries, passionfruit pulp and coconut. Cut into wedges to serve immediately.

PER SERVE 2.7g protein, 2.5g fat (0.4g saturated fat), 65.9g carb, 1.6g dietary fibre, 292 Cals (1222kJ)

make it your way

SHOP FROZEN If mangoes and raspberries aren't in season, buy the fruit frozen. Simply thaw before decorating the cake. You can also use other fresh fruit, such as banana, to decorate, if you like.

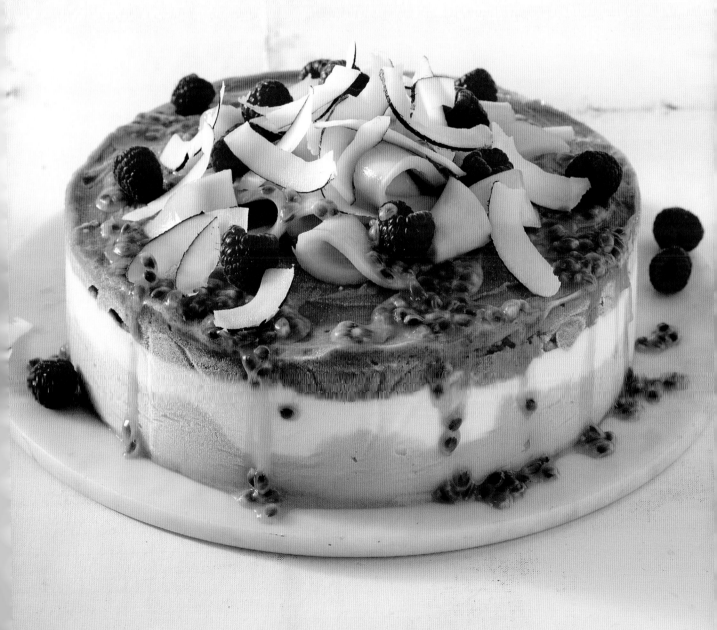

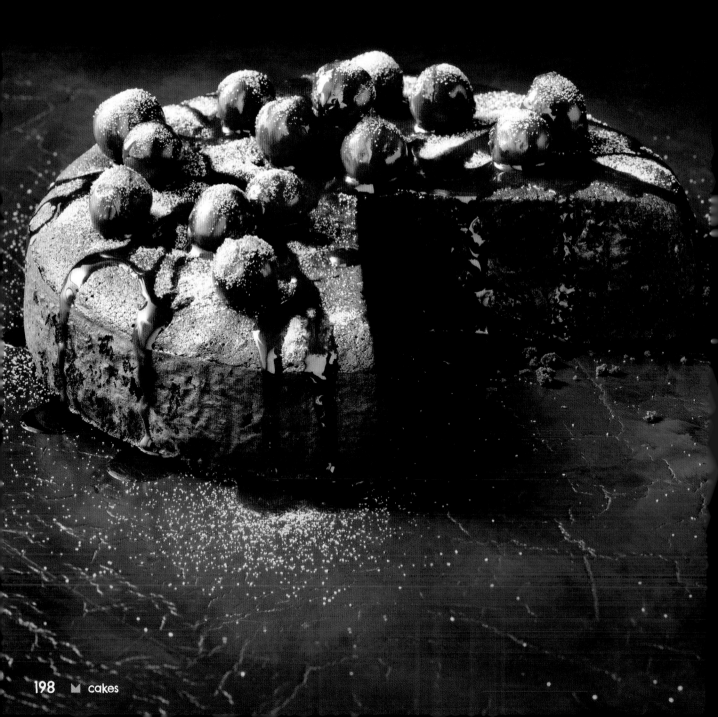

chocolate cherry CAKE

This wonderfully dense cake is gluten free and has just the right amount of chocolatey sweetness to complement the tartness of Morello cherries.

serves 8   **prep** 30 mins (+ cooling & 1 hour chilling)   **cook** 40 mins

ingredients

50g dark chocolate
  (85% cocoa), chopped
2 tbs coconut oil
210g coconut syrup or
  maple syrup
125ml (½ cup) Morello
  sour cherry juice
80ml (⅓ cup) brandy
100g (1 cup) almond meal
35g (⅓ cup) raw cacao powder,
  plus 2 tbs extra
40g (¼ cup) buckwheat flour
½ tsp gluten-free baking powder
3 eggs, separated
110g (½ cup) Morello sour
  cherries, drained, plus
  extra, to serve
50g coconut sugar
Edible glitter, to serve (optional)

1 Preheat oven to 180°C/160°C fan forced. Grease the base and side of a 20cm (base size) springform pan and line with baking paper. Place the chocolate, oil, 115g syrup, 60ml (¼ cup) cherry juice and 2 tbs brandy in a saucepan over medium heat. Cook, stirring, for 3 minutes or until smooth. Transfer to a bowl.

2 Stir the almond meal, cacao, flour, baking powder, yolks and cherries into the chocolate mixture. Use electric beaters to beat the egg whites in a bowl until stiff peaks form. Slowly add sugar, beating until thick.

3 Fold half the egg white into the chocolate mixture. Fold in remaining egg white until just combined. Pour into prepared pan. Bake for 30 minutes or until a skewer inserted into the centre comes out clean. Cool in pan for 15 minutes. Transfer to a wire rack to cool completely.

4 Whisk remaining syrup, juice, brandy and extra cacao in a saucepan over medium-low heat for 1 minute or until smooth. Bring to the boil. Simmer for 3-4 minutes. Cool. Place in fridge for 1 hour to thicken. Top cake with extra cherries, brandy sauce and glitter, if using. Serve.

PER SERVE 7.2g protein, 14g fat (5.7g saturated fat), 45.5g carb, 5.1g dietary fibre, 348 Cals (1454kJ)

TRY Serve the cake with a large dollop of whipped dairy-free cream or spoonfuls of coconut yoghurt, if you like.

strawberry 'milkshake' CAKE

EF DF NF SF SBF FSF

We've taken the strawberry and vanilla creaminess of a milkshake and turned it into a party cake without egg, milk or butter.

serves 30 **prep** 45 mins (+ cooling) **cook** 50 mins

ingredients

675g (4½ cups) plain flour
315g (1½) cups caster sugar
375ml (1½ cups) sunflower oil
1 tbs vanilla extract
500ml (2 cups) rice milk
3 tsp bicarbonate of soda
60ml (¼ cup) apple cider vinegar
½ x 200g bag pink and white
    marshmallow puffs
½ x 170g bag milk bottle lollies
12 jubes, halved
2 tbs mixed star sprinkles

strawberry frosting

375g Nuttelex spread
675g (4½ cups) pure icing sugar
2 tsp Queen Strawb'ry & Cream
    Flavour for Icing
Pink gel food colouring, to tint

1 Preheat oven to 180°C/160°C fan forced. Grease a 20 x 30cm (base size) lamington pan. Line with baking paper, extending paper 5cm above edges. Combine 340g (2¼ cups) flour and 155g (¾ cup) sugar in a bowl. Make a well. Add 180ml (¾ cup) oil and 2 tsp vanilla to well (don't stir). Place 250ml (1 cup) rice milk in a jug. Add 1½ tsp bicarb and 1½ tbs vinegar. Whisk until frothy. Add to well. Stir until smooth and combined. Spoon into prepared pan. Smooth the surface.

2 Bake cake for 25 minutes or until a skewer inserted into the centre comes out clean. Cool in pan for 10 minutes. Transfer, top-side up, onto a wire rack to cool completely. Repeat step 1 for a second cake.

3 To make frosting, use an electric mixer to beat Nuttelex and icing sugar until light and fluffy. Beat in flavouring. Tint pink with food colouring.

4 Spoon 1 cup frosting into a sealable bag and snip off 1 corner. Place 1 cake on a board. Spread with 1 cup remaining frosting. Top with second cake. Spread top and sides with remaining frosting. Pipe small swirls on top. Top with sweets. Decorate with sprinkles. Serve.

PER SERVE 2.6g protein, 20.2g fat (4.2g saturated fat), 56.3g carb, 0.8g dietary fibre, 412 Cals (1723kJ)

make it your way

CHANGE IT UP Top with your favourite soft sweets. Try strawberries & cream lollies (contain wheat) and halved lolly raspberries.

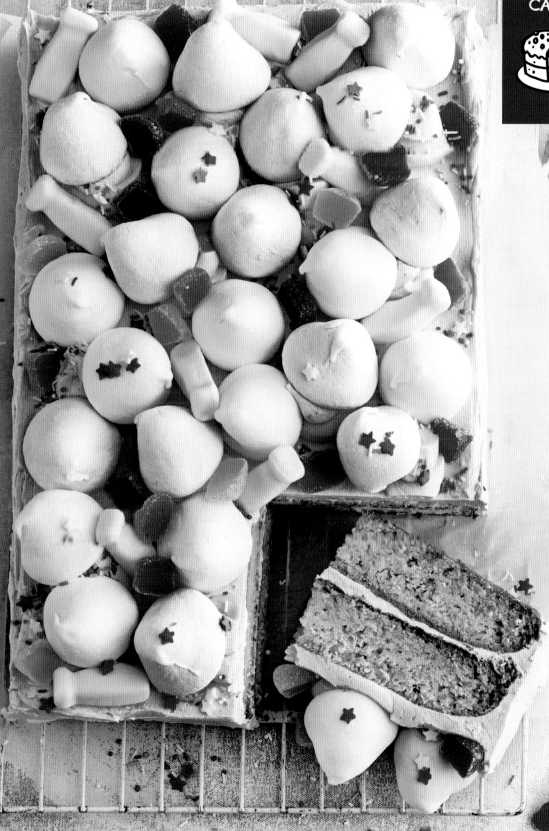

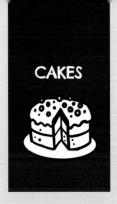

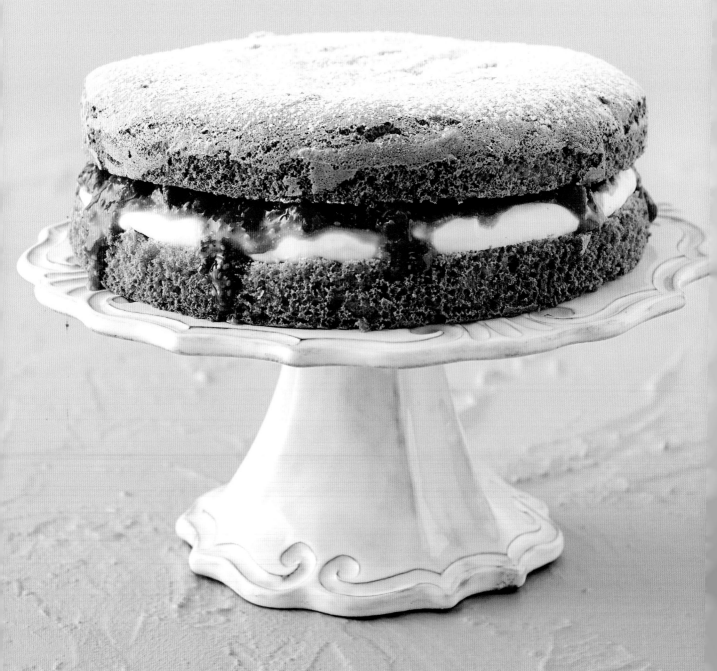

coconut + strawberry
SPONGE

DF NF SF GF SBF FSF

The perfect dairy- and gluten-free sponge to enjoy with a steaming hot cuppa and good conversation.

serves 8   **prep** 30 mins (+ cooling, standing & chilling)   **cook** 30 mins

ingredients

3 eggs, separated
2½ tbs caster sugar
40g (¼ cup) coconut sugar
½ tsp vanilla extract
70g (½ cup) gluten-free cornflour
45g (¼ cup) brown rice flour
¾ tsp cream of tartar
½ tsp bicarbonate of soda
1 tbs fine desiccated coconut
250g strawberries, hulled, chopped
1 tbs lemon juice
1½ tsp chia seeds
½ tsp vanilla bean paste
270ml can coconut milk, chilled for 4-6 hours
Pure icing sugar, to dust

1 Preheat oven to 180°C/160°C fan forced. Grease base and side of a 6cm-deep, 20cm (base size) round cake pan. Line with baking paper. Use electric beaters to beat egg whites in a bowl for 1 minute or until frothy. Combine caster sugar and 2 tbs coconut sugar in a bowl. Add to egg white, 1 tbs at a time, beating well after each addition. Beat for 2 minutes or until tripled in volume. Add yolks, 1 at a time, beating well after each addition. Beat in vanilla. Sift flours, cream of tartar and bicarb into bowl. Add coconut. Gently fold until just combined. Spoon into prepared pan. Bake for 20-22 minutes or until springs back when lightly touched. Cool in pan for 5 minutes. Turn onto a wire rack to cool.

2 Meanwhile, place strawberry, lemon juice and remaining coconut sugar in a saucepan. Cook, stirring, over low heat for 7 minutes or until strawberry breaks down. Stir in chia seeds for 1 minute or until thick. Transfer to a bowl. Cool for 30 minutes. Place in fridge for 30 minutes.

3 Spoon solid coconut milk from can into a bowl (discard liquid). Add vanilla. Whisk until thick. Halve cake in horizontally. Top with coconut cream and strawberry mix. Add cake top. Dust with icing sugar. Serve.

PER SERVE 3.9g protein, 8.1g fat (5.9g saturated fat), 24.2g carb, 0.9g dietary fibre, 184 Cals (770kJ)

make it your way

BOOST Turn this sponge into a celebration cake by making another batch of coconut cream for the top and decorating with fresh berries.

chocolate, hazelnut +
PEAR CAKE

DF SF GF SBF FSF

Studded with slices of fresh pear and chunks of dark chocolate, this wholesome cake is free of gluten, dairy and refined sugar.

serves 12   **prep** 30 mins (+ cooling)   **cook** 1 hour

ingredients

4 eggs, separated
75g (⅓ cup) Natvia for Baking
80ml (⅓ cup) honey
2 tsp vanilla extract
125ml (½ cup) light extra
   virgin olive oil
140g (1⅓ cups) hazelnut meal
35g (⅓ cup) desiccated coconut
35g (⅓ cup) raw cacao powder
40g (¼ cup) buckwheat flour
2 (about 450g) just-ripe pears,
   cored, thinly sliced
100g dark chocolate
   (85% cocoa), chopped
1 tbs chopped hazelnuts

1 Preheat oven to 180°C/160°C fan forced. Grease base and side of a 22cm round springform cake pan. Line with baking paper. Use electric beaters to beat egg yolks, Natvia, honey and vanilla in a bowl for 5 minutes or until doubled in size and a ribbon trail forms when beater is lifted. Add the oil in a steady stream, beating until thick.

2 Combine hazelnut meal, coconut, cacao and flour in a bowl. Use clean electric beaters to beat egg whites in a separate bowl until firm peaks form. In 2 batches, use a metal spoon to fold hazelnut mixture and egg white into the yolk mixture until just combined. Pour half the batter into prepared pan. Top with half the pear and chocolate. Pour over remaining batter. Top with the remaining pear, arranging in a concentric circle. Sprinkle with hazelnut and remaining chocolate.

3 Bake for 50-60 minutes or until a skewer inserted into the cake comes out clean. Cool in pan for 15 minutes. Transfer to a wire rack to cool completely. Serve.

PER SERVE 6g protein, 25g fat (6g saturated fat), 14g carb, 4g dietary fibre, 336 Cals (1365kJ)

make it your way

DAIRY ADDED? If concerned with dairy contamination in the dark chocolate, opt for soy-based dark chocolate (contains soy).
BOOST Serve the cake with whipped dairy-free cream.

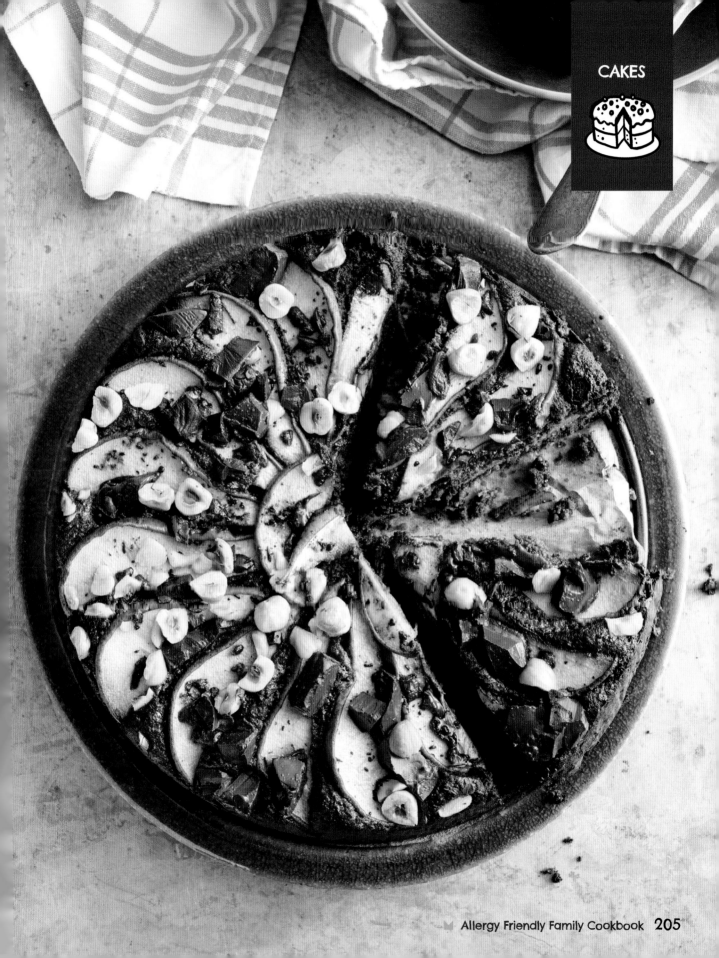

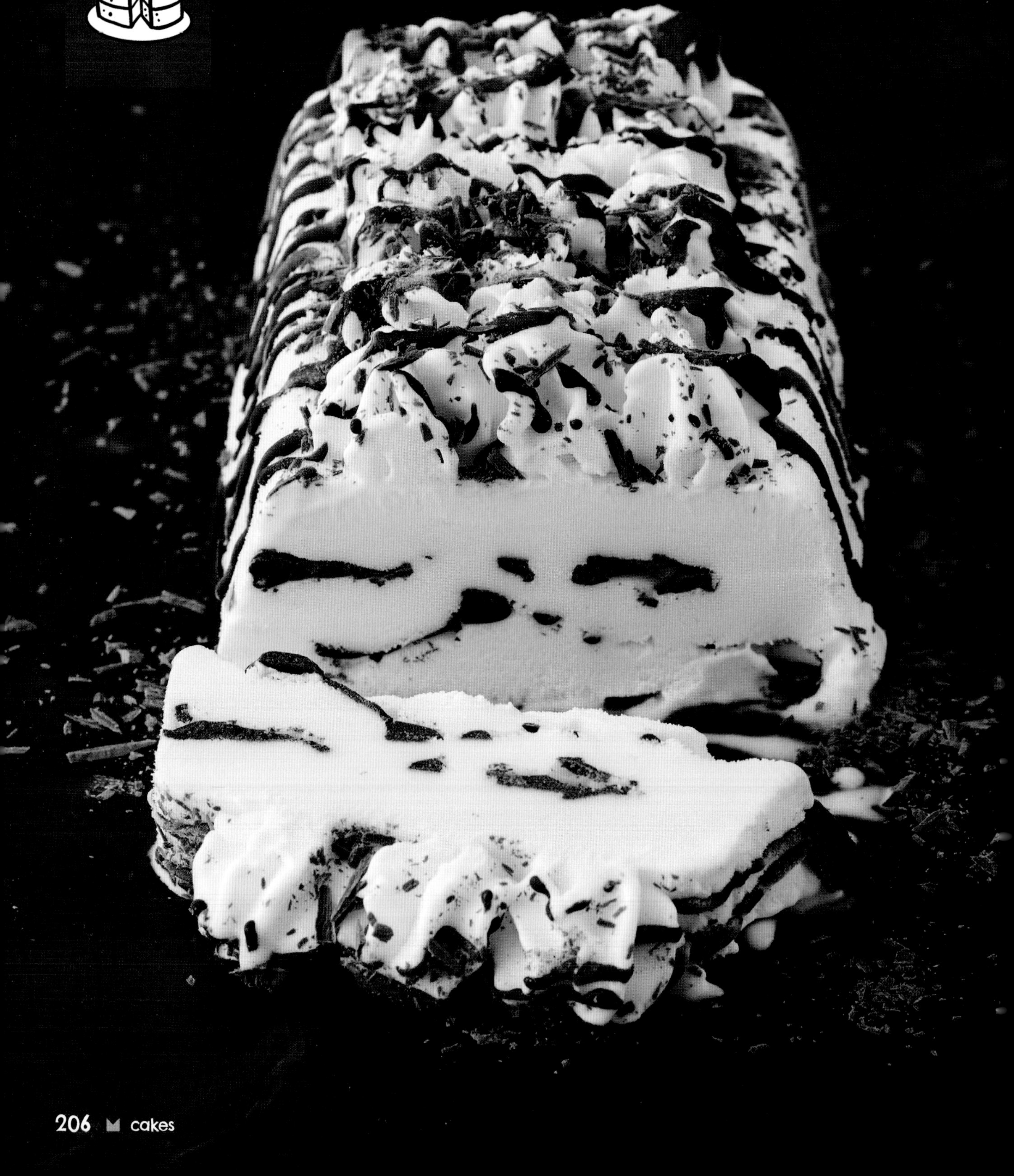

choc-coconut VEGANETTA

Pass your childhood love of Vienetta down to your kids with this vegan version of the popular retro ice-cream.

serves 8 **prep** 25 mins (+ 3 hours 10 mins freezing)

ingredients
60g (¼ cup) solid coconut oil
30g (¼ cup) cacao powder
2 tbs maple syrup
1L vegan coconut ice-cream
Coarsely grated dairy-free chocolate, to serve

1 Combine the oil, cacao and syrup in a microwave-safe bowl. Microwave for 15 seconds or until oil is melted. Stir until smooth.

2 Lightly grease the base of a 9 x 19cm (base size) loaf pan with oil. Line with baking paper, allowing the 2 long sides to overhang. Use a dessert spoon to scoop out one-quarter of the ice-cream in flat pieces and use to cover base of prepared pan. Return remaining ice-cream to freezer. Gently press and smooth the surface. Drizzle with 2 tbs cacao mixture. Place in freezer for 1 hour or until firm. Repeat to make 2 more layers of ice-cream and cacao mixture.

3 Turn ice-cream loaf onto a chilled serving platter. Return to freezer. Scoop remaining ice-cream into a piping bag fitted with a large fluted or star nozzle. Stand at room temperature for a few minutes or until soft but not melted. Pipe rosettes over top of loaf. Return to the freezer for 5 minutes or until firm.

4 Drizzle remaining cacao mixture over ice-cream loaf. Freeze for 5 minutes or until firm. Sprinkle with chocolate. Slice, to serve.

PER SERVE 1.9g protein, 21.3g fat (18.1g saturated fat), 13.7g carb, 1.2g dietary fibre, 236 Cals (987kJ)

make it your way

BOOST Drizzle a little vegan caramel sauce over each layer of ice-cream and cacao mixture before freezing.

community recipe
chocolate birthday
CUPCAKES

EF · DF · SF · SBF · FSF

"These cupcakes are great to have on hand in the freezer. You can make them up to 1 month ahead of time. Simply defrost to take to a party as an allergy-friendly treat." ~ *Catherine Hornung*

makes 15   **prep** 30 mins (+ cooling)   **cook** 25 mins

ingredients

200g (1⅓ cups) plain flour
70g (⅔ cup) cocoa powder
1 tsp bicarbonate of soda
1 tsp baking powder
155g (¾ cup) caster sugar
250ml (1 cup) dairy- and
 soy-free milk
1 tsp white vinegar
250g (1 cup) apple sauce
125g (½ cup) Nuttelex, melted
1 tsp vanilla extract

choc frosting

50g dairy- and soy-free
 chocolate buttons
60ml (¼ cup) almond milk
380g (2½ cups) icing sugar mixture
70g (⅔ cup) cocoa powder
250g (1 cup) Nuttelex spread
2 tsp vanilla extract

1 Preheat oven to 170°C/150°C fan forced. Line 15 x 80ml (⅓ cup) muffin pans with paper cases. Sift flour, cocoa powder, bicarb, baking powder and a pinch of salt into a bowl. Stir in sugar. Make a well. Whisk milk with vinegar in a jug. Stir in apple sauce, Nuttelex, 80ml (⅓ cup) water and vanilla. Add to well. Fold to combine. Divide between muffin pans.

2 Bake for 20-25 minutes or until cupcakes are springy to a gentle touch. Cool in pan for 5 minutes. Transfer to a wire rack to cool completely.

3 To make the frosting, combine the chocolate and milk in a small bowl. Microwave, stirring halfway, for 1 minute. Stir until smooth. Let cool.

4 Sift the icing sugar and cocoa into a bowl. Use electric beaters to beat the Nuttelex and vanilla in a bowl until combined. Add icing sugar, 1 large spoonful at a time, beating after each addition, until light and fluffy. Beat in cooled chocolate mixture. Pipe or spread frosting onto cupcakes, to serve.

PER SERVE 3.3g protein, 19.4g fat (5.8g saturated fat), 49.5g carb, 3.3g dietary fibre, 384 Cals (1608kJ)

 make it your way NUT FREE Instead of almond milk, choose a nut-free, plant-based milk. FREEZE IT Cupcakes can be frozen with or without frosting.

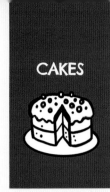

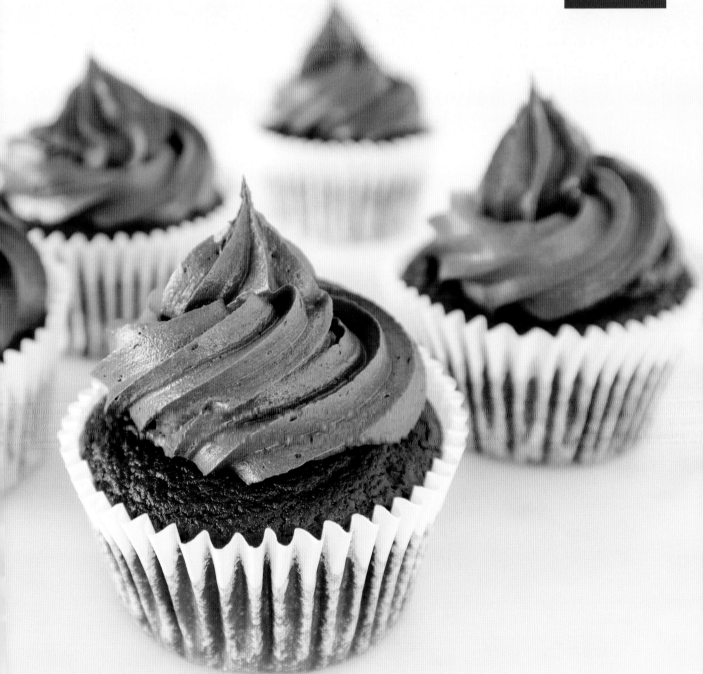

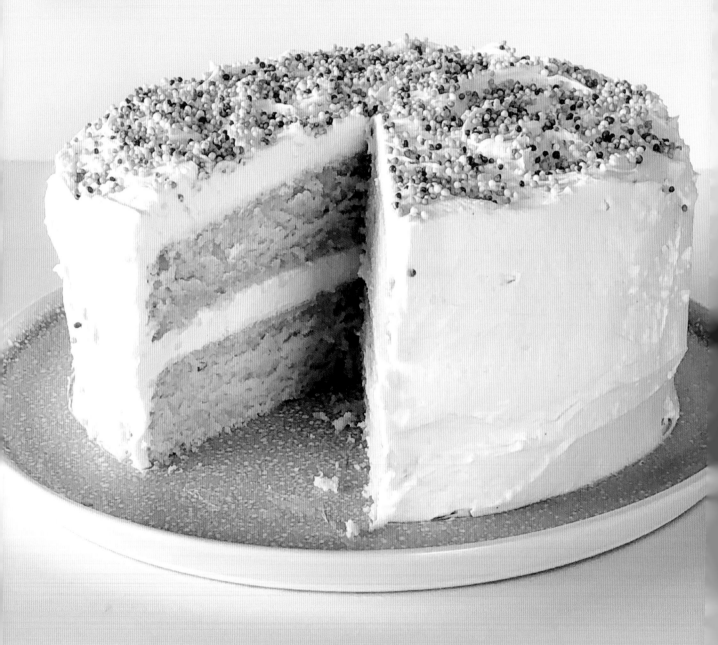

community recipe
vanilla birthday
CAKE

EF   DF   NF   SF   SBF   FSF

"Twenty-five years ago, I was looking for an egg-free cake that I could make for my children, two of whom had an egg and nut allergy. I came across a recipe and adapted it to this cake over the years. It can be decorated and coloured to your liking." ~ *Kristen Cousins*

serves 12   **prep** 30 mins (+ cooling)   **cook** 35 mins

ingredients
2 tbs vegetable oil
4½ tsp baking powder
450g (3 cups) plain flour
370g (1¾ cups) caster sugar
½ tsp vanilla extract
125g (½ cup) Nuttelex spread
Sprinkles, to decorate

creamy vanilla frosting
375g (1½ cups) Nuttelex spread
600g (4 cups) icing
   sugar mixture
2 tbs hot water
1 tsp vanilla extract

1 Preheat oven to 180°C/160°C fan forced. Grease two 20cm (base size) round cake pans. Line bases with baking paper. Use electric beaters to beat the oil, 60ml (¼ cup) water and baking powder on low speed for 30 seconds or until combined. Add remaining ingredients and 310ml (1¼ cups) water. Beat for 1 minute. Increase speed to medium. Beat for 3 minutes or until thickened. Divide among prepared pans.

2 Bake for 35 minutes or until a skewer inserted into centre of the cakes comes out clean. Cool in pans for 5 minutes. Turn onto a wire rack top-side up to cool completely.

3 To make the frosting, use electric beaters on medium-high speed to beat the Nuttelex until light and fluffy. Gradually add icing sugar, beating until combined. Beat in water and vanilla until just combined. Place 1 cake on a cake plate. Spread with one-third of the frosting. Top with second cake. Spread top and side with remaining frosting. Decorate with sprinkles, to serve.

PER SERVE 3.8g protein, 23.9g fat (5.9g saturated fat), 109.8g carb, 0.8g dietary fibre, 657 Cals (2748kJ)

make it your way

BOOST Decorate cake with grated vegan chocolate (may contain soy). Or add a little food colouring to tint frosting your favourite colour.

community recipe
lauren's
CHEESECAKE

EF DF NF SF GF FSF

*"Cheesecake is always a welcome dessert cake.
This vegan option is delightfully light and the fresh
seasonal raspberries add a delicious tang."* ~ Frances Oppedisano

serves 8   **prep** 30 mins (+ 4 hours 15 mins chilling)   **cook** 40 mins

ingredients

180g gluten-free digestive
   biscuits, crushed
70g (⅓ cup) caster sugar
½ tsp ground cinnamon
80g (⅓ cup) dairy-free
   margarine, melted

filling

450g vegan cream cheese, at
   room temperature, chopped
140g (⅔ cup) caster sugar
2 tbs cornflour
60ml (¼ cup) oat milk
1 tbs fresh lemon juice
1 tsp vanilla bean paste
125g fresh raspberries
Pure icing sugar, to dust

1 Preheat oven to 180°C/160°C fan forced. Grease an 18cm round springform pan. Line the base with baking paper.

2 Combine the biscuit, sugar, cinnamon and margarine in a bowl. Press mixture over the base and halfway up the side of the prepared pan. Place in the fridge for 15 minutes or until firm.

3 To make the filling, use electric beaters to beat the cream cheese and sugar in a bowl until smooth and creamy. Combine cornflour and milk in a jug until smooth. Add to cream cheese mixture with lemon juice and vanilla. Beat until combined and smooth. Pour over biscuit base.

4 Stand pan on a baking tray. Bake for 40 minutes or until set but a bit wobbly. Cool completely. Place in fridge for 4 hours, or overnight.

5 Arrange the fresh raspberries over the top of the cheesecake and dust lightly with icing sugar, to serve.

PER SERVE 5.6g protein, 28g fat (17.6g saturated fat), 45.3g carb, 4g dietary fibre, 455 Cals (1905kJ)

make it your way

BOOST Drizzle top of cheesecake with vegan caramel sauce, spread with passionfruit pulp, or grate over soy-free vegan chocolate.

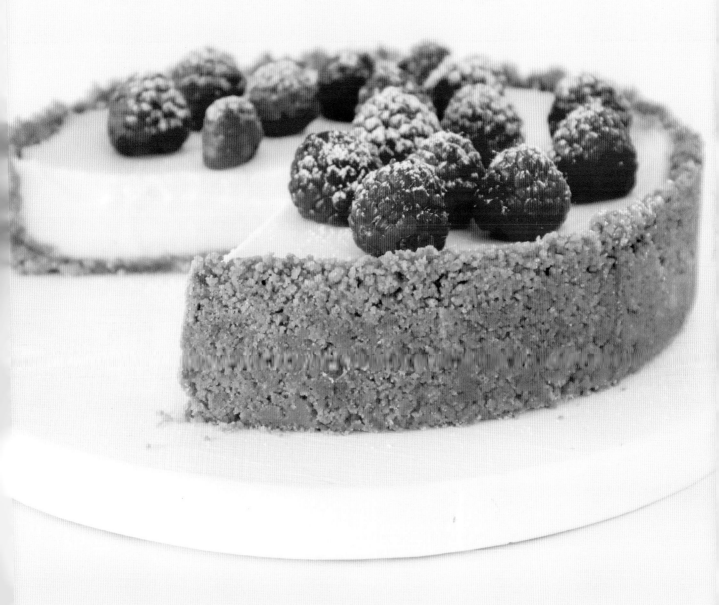

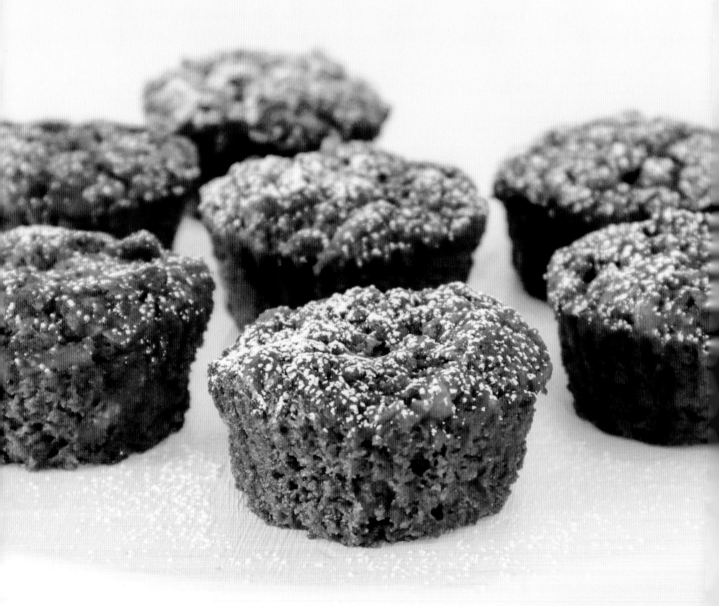

community recipe
carrot + ginger
CUPCAKES

EF DF NF SF SBF FSF

"These are my favourite allergy-free cakes for birthday parties, bake sales and afternoon munchies. My son has anaphylaxis to dairy, egg and nuts, which makes it difficult for him at parties. We take along a plate of these and they disappear quickly!" ~ *Sarah MacFarlane*

makes 16   **prep** 20 mins (+ cooling)   **cook** 20 mins

ingredients

250g (about 2 carrots), peeled, grated
160ml (⅔ cup) sunflower oil
125g (¾ cup, lightly packed) dark brown sugar
150g (1 cup) plain flour
1 tsp ground cinnamon
2 tsp ground ginger
1 tsp bicarbonate of soda
½ tsp baking powder
¼ tsp salt
2 tsp egg replacer
Pure icing sugar, to dust

1 Preheat oven to 180°C/160°C fan forced. Lightly grease 16 x 50ml cupcake pans with oil. Combine the carrot, oil and sugar in a large bowl. Sift the flour, cinnamon, ginger, bicarb, baking powder and salt into the bowl. Fold in until evenly combined.

2 Combine egg replacer and 60ml (¼ cup) water in a small bowl. Add to carrot mixture and fold through until just combined (don't over mix).

3 Divide batter evenly among the cupcake pans. Bake for 20 minutes or until springy to a gentle touch. Cool cakes in the pan for 5 minutes before transferring to a wire rack to cool completely. Dust lightly with icing sugar, to serve.

PER SERVE 1.1g protein, 9.4g fat (1g saturated fat), 15.9g carb, 0.9g dietary fibre, 152 Cals (634kJ)

make it your way

FROST IT Use electric beaters to whip 125g dairy-free cream cheese, 230g (1½ cups) pure icing sugar and 1 tsp vanilla extract in a bowl until light and fluffy. Spread over cupcakes.

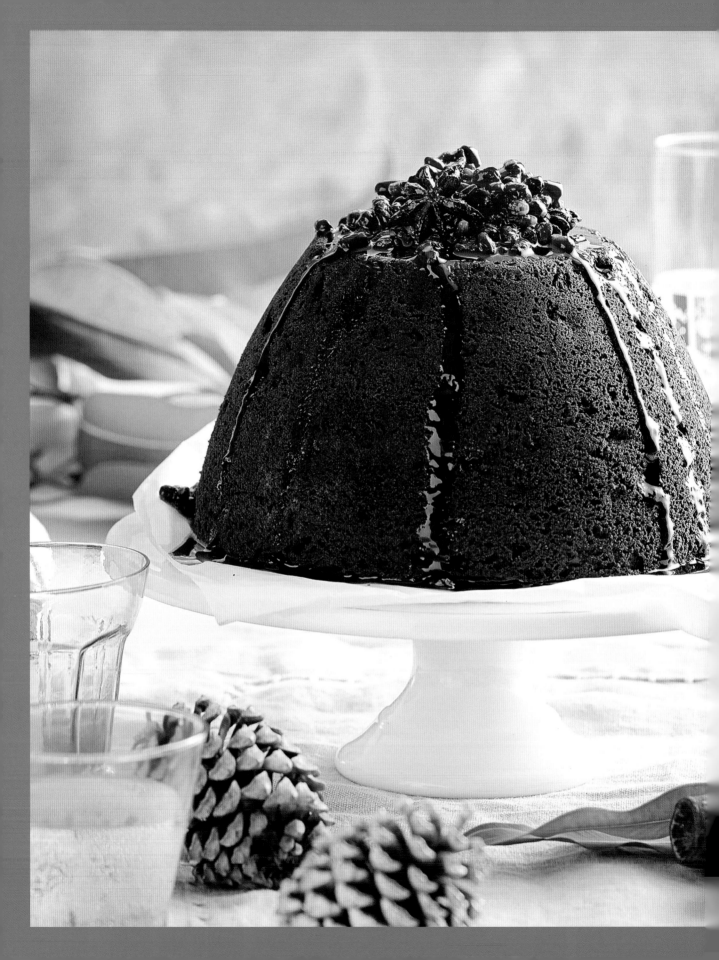

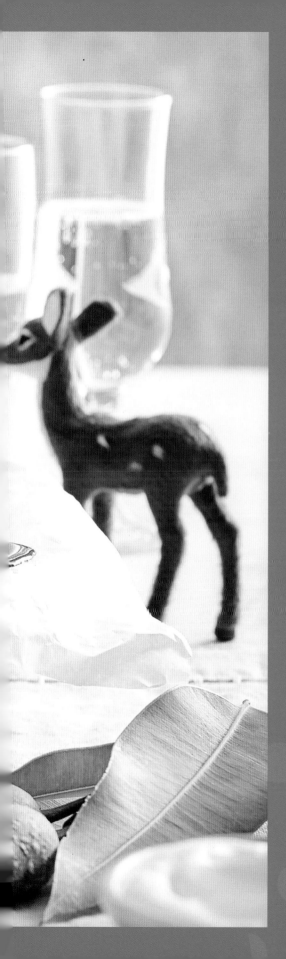

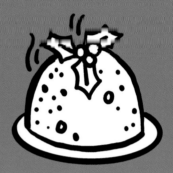

celebrate traditions

We've made celebrating easy with an inclusive collection of allergy-friendly recipes.

gluten-free hot cross BUNS

 NF SF GF SBF FSF

Hot cross buns aren't just for Easter. Make these sweet buns all year with this gluten-free version.

makes 20   **prep** 30 mins (+ 15 mins cooling & 1 hour standing)   **cook** 35 mins

ingredients

250ml (1 cup) milk
100g (½ cup) caster sugar
100g butter, chopped
110g (⅔ cup) mixed dried fruit
280g (2 cups) buckwheat flour, plus extra, to dust
270g (1½ cups) brown rice flour, plus extra 90g (½ cup)
130g (1 cup) tapioca flour
2 tsp xanthan gum
2 x 7g sachets dried yeast
2 tsp ground cinnamon
½ tsp ground nutmeg
½ tsp allspice
¼ tsp ground cloves
2 eggs, lightly whisked
5 tbs cold water
2 tbs honey, warmed
Butter, to serve

1 Place the milk, sugar, butter and dried fruit in a saucepan over medium heat. Cook, stirring occasionally, for 5 minutes or until mixture is almost simmering. Remove from heat. Cool for 15 minutes.

2 Meanwhile, combine flours, xanthan gum, yeast and spices in a large bowl. Make a well. Add milk mixture and egg to well. Stir until a dough forms. Turn out onto a lightly floured surface. Knead for 10 minutes or until smooth. Place dough in a lightly oiled bowl. Cover with greased plastic wrap. Stand in a warm place for 1 hour or until doubled in size.

3 Preheat oven to 200°C/180°C fan forced. Line a large baking tray with baking paper. Divide dough into 20 balls. Use picture as a guide to arrange dough balls in a circle on prepared tray. Cover with a clean tea towel. Set aside for 30 minutes or until buns have risen slightly.

4 Make a thin paste by combining extra brown rice flour and cold water. Transfer to a sealable bag. Snip off 1 corner. Pipe crosses on top of each bun. Bake for 20 minutes or until starting to brown. Gently brush tops with honey. Bake for 5-10 minutes or until golden. Serve with butter.

PER SERVE 4.1g protein, 5.9g fat (3.4g saturated fat), 37.7g carb, 2.6g dietary fibre, 224 Cals (938kJ)

make it your way

DAIRY FREE Use soy (contains soy) or oat milk in place of regular milk, and use a plant-based butter for cooking and spreading.

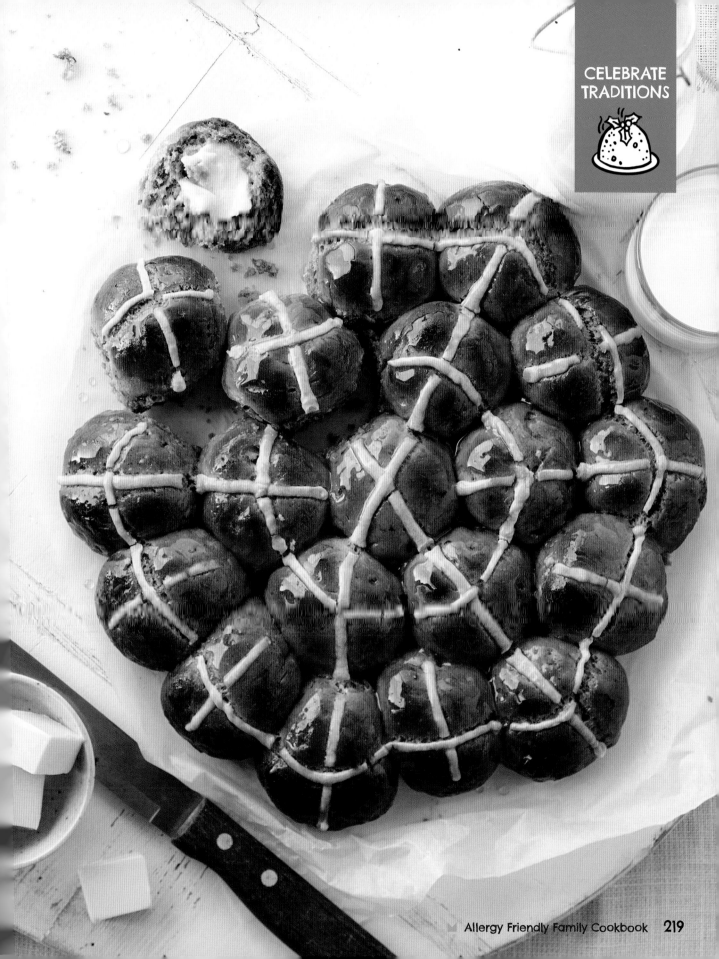

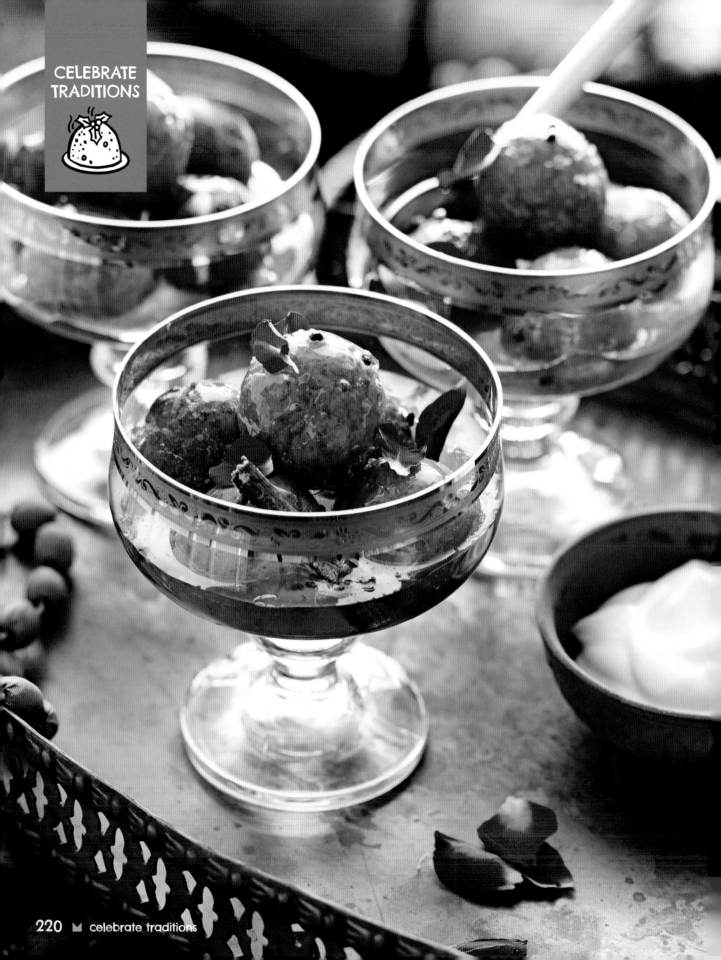

gulab JAMUN

EF NF SF SBF FSF

Quick and easy to prepare, this irresistibly sweet, syrupy dessert is perfect for Eid and other Islamic festivities.

serves 6   **prep** 20 mins (+ cooling & 30 mins soaking)   **cook** 20 mins

ingredients

430g (2 cups) caster sugar
1 cinnamon stick
1 tsp cardamom seeds
¼ tsp rosewater essence
120g (1 cup) full-cream
    milk powder
75g (½ cup) self-raising flour
¼ tsp bicarbonate of soda
1 tsp ground cardamom
25g butter, chopped
500ml (2 cups) vegetable oil
Greek-style natural yoghurt
    and rose petals (optional),
    to serve

1 Combine 500ml (2 cups) water, sugar, cinnamon and cardamom seeds in a saucepan over medium-high heat. Stir until sugar dissolves. Simmer for 5 minutes or until slightly thick. Stir in rosewater. Cool slightly.

2 Combine the milk powder, flour, bicarb and ground cardamom in a bowl. Use your fingertips to rub the butter into the flour. Add 80ml (⅓ cup) water, a little at a time, until dough is soft and sticky. Shape heaped teaspoonfuls of dough into balls. Place on a large tray.

3 Heat the oil in a large wok or saucepan over high heat until 170°C on a cook's thermomoter (or when a cube of bread turns golden in 20 seconds). Reduce heat to low. Cook one-third of the balls, turning occasionally, for 2 minutes or until golden and cooked through. Transfer to a tray lined with paper towel. Repeat with remaining balls, in 2 more batches, reheating oil and reducing heat to low between batches.

4 Arrange balls in a single layer in a deep dish. Pour over syrup. Stand for 30 minutes to soak. Serve with yoghurt and rose petals, if using.

PER SERVE 6.5g protein, 48g fat (9.5g saturated fat), 88g carb, 0.5g dietary fibre, 796 Cals (3330kJ)

make it your way

DAIRY FREE Swap milk powder for soy milk powder (contains soy) or coconut milk powder, and use dairy-free butter and coconut yoghurt.

berry + cherry
SUMMER PUDS

When a hot Aussie summer Yule is on the cards, these gorgeous puddings make a great finale to lunch or dinner.

makes 6   prep 45 mins (+ cooling & overnight chilling)   cook 10 mins

ingredients

250g punnet strawberries, hulled, chopped
125g punnet raspberries
250g frozen mixed berries
250g fresh cherries, pitted, chopped
75g (⅓ cup) raw sugar
1 vanilla bean, split
1 orange, rind finely grated, juiced
520g loaf thickly sliced gluten-free white bread, crusts removed, slices halved horizontally and flattened with a rolling pin
Extra fresh berries, edible flowers (optional) and coconut yoghurt, to serve

1 Lightly spray six 5.5cm (base size), 7.5cm (top size), 125ml (½ cup) round moulds with oil. Combine berries and cherries in a saucepan. Add the sugar, vanilla bean, orange rind, 125ml (½ cup) orange juice and 160ml (⅔ cup) water. Cook, stirring, over medium heat until the sugar dissolves. Bring to the boil. Simmer for 3-5 minutes or until thickened slightly. Cool completely. Strain, reserving berries and liquid.

2 Use round 5.5cm and 7.5cm cutters to cut out 6 rounds each from bread slices. Discard scraps. Halve remaining slices crossways.

3 Dip smaller rounds into reserved berry liquid. Place 1 round in the base of each mould. Dip halved bread slices in berry liquid. Firmly press 3 around the edge of each mould, overlapping slightly. Fill moulds with reserved berries, packing tightly. Dip larger bread rounds in remaining berry liquid. Place on moulds. Reserve any remaining liquid. Cover tightly with plastic wrap. Place in fridge overnight to chill.

4 Turn puddings onto plates. Top with reserved berry liquid, extra fresh berries and flowers, if using. Serve with coconut yoghurt.

PER SERVE 8g protein, 5g fat (1g saturated fat), 60g carb, 9g dietary fibre, 335 Cals (1403kJ)

make it your way

MAKE AHEAD Make puds 1-2 days ahead of serving to infuse flavours.
NOTE Gluten-free bread may contain soy, nuts, egg and dairy

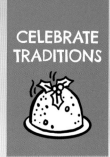

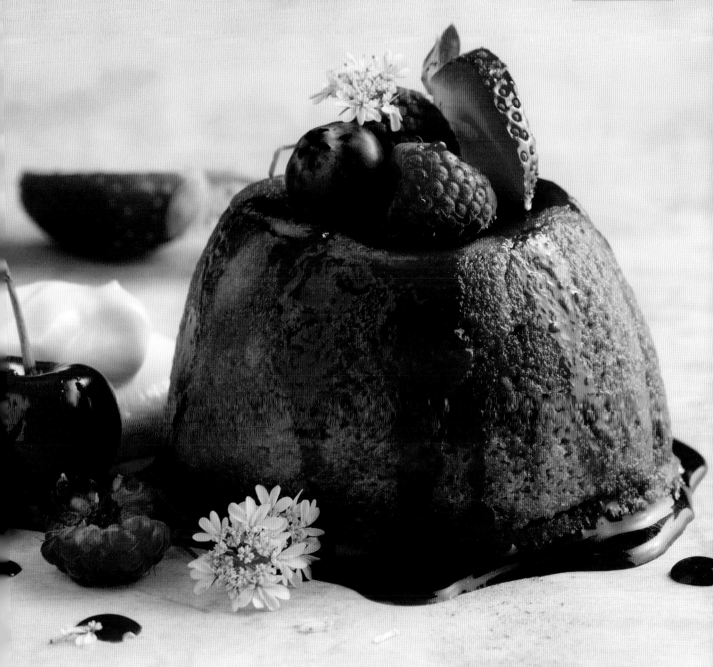

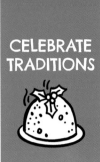

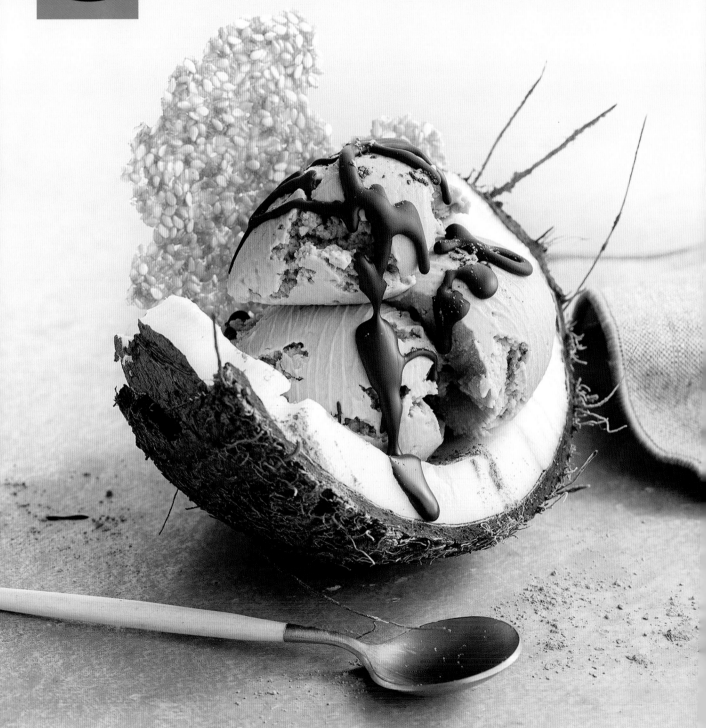

green goddess
SUNDAE

This dessert not only looks spectacular, it will bring smiles all round this coming Chinese New Year.

makes 4   **prep** 30 mins (+ cooling & 12 hours freezing)   **cook** 10 mins

ingredients
1 large mature coconut, broken
   into 4 large pieces
80g 70% cocoa dark
   chocolate, melted
Matcha powder, to sprinkle

coconut matcha ice cream
400ml can coconut cream
80ml (⅓ cup) honey
70g avocado flesh
2-3 tsp matcha powder

sesame coconut brittle
2 tbs sesame seeds
2 tsp desiccated coconut
1½ tbs honey

1 To make the ice-cream, pour the coconut cream into ice cube trays and place in the freezer for 8 hours, or overnight, until frozen.

2 Meanwhile, to make the coconut brittle, preheat oven to 180°C/160°C fan forced. Line a baking tray with baking paper. Place sesame seeds, coconut and honey in a microwave-safe bowl. Microwave for 30 seconds. Stir to combine. Spread over prepared tray. Bake for 8 minutes or until dark golden. Cool. Break into large shards.

3 Use a blender to blend the frozen coconut cream and honey, scraping down side with a spatula as needed, for 1 minute or until smooth and combined. Add avocado and matcha powder. Blend for 1-2 minutes or until smooth and creamy. Transfer to an airtight container and place in the freezer for 4 hours or until firm.

4 Just before serving, place 2 scoops of ice-cream into each coconut 'bowl'. Drizzle with melted chocolate. Top with shards of sesame brittle and sprinkle with extra matcha powder, to serve.

PER SERVE 5g protein, 35g fat (24g saturated fat), 45g carb,
2g dietary fibre, 511 Cals (2138kJ)

make it your way

SOY FREE Opt for soy-free dark chocolate (may contain dairy).
SESAME FREE Omit the sesame seeds or replace with flaxseeds.

nut-free fruity
BAKLAVA

Diwali's festival of lights wouldn't be complete without diamonds of homemade baklava. Our nut-free take is divine!

serves 16   prep 10 mins   cook 45 mins

ingredients

85g (1 cup) desiccated coconut
135g (¾ cup) dried apricots, chopped
125g (¾ cup) currants
55g (¼ cup) caster sugar
½ tsp ground cinnamon
15 sheets filo pastry
200g unsalted butter, melted

spiced syrup
1 tbs honey
½ tsp ground cinnamon
1 tsp finely grated orange rind
215g (1 cup) caster sugar
160ml (⅔ cup) cold water

1 Preheat oven to 180°C/160°C fan forced. Grease a 20 x 30cm (base size) lamington pan. Process coconut, apricot and currants in a food processor until finely chopped. Stir in sugar and cinnamon.

2 Brush 1 sheet pastry with melted butter. Top with another sheet and brush with melted butter. Fold sheets in half. Press into prepared pan. Sprinkle with ½ cup coconut mixture. Brush 1 sheet pastry with melted butter. Fold in half. Place on top of coconut mixture. Sprinkle with 2 tbs coconut mixture. Continue layering, finishing with pastry.

3 Using a sharp knife, trim edges. Cut baklava layers into thirds lengthways, then crossways diagonally, to make 16 diamond-shaped pieces. Bake for 30 minutes. Reduce heat to 150°C/130°C fan forced. Bake for a further 10-15 minutes or until golden.

4 Meanwhile, to make the syrup, place all ingredients in a saucepan over medium-high heat. Cook, stirring, until sugar dissolves. Bring to the boil. Reduce heat to medium. Simmer for 5 minutes or until has slightly thickened. Pour syrup over hot baklava. Cool in pan. Serve.

PER SERVE 2.1g protein, 12.2g fat (8.6g saturated fat), 32.7g carb, 2.1g dietary fibre, 240 Cals (1000kJ)

make it your way

DAIRY FREE Opt for a plant-based unsalted butter.
ADULTS ONLY Serve the baklava with a strong cup of black coffee.

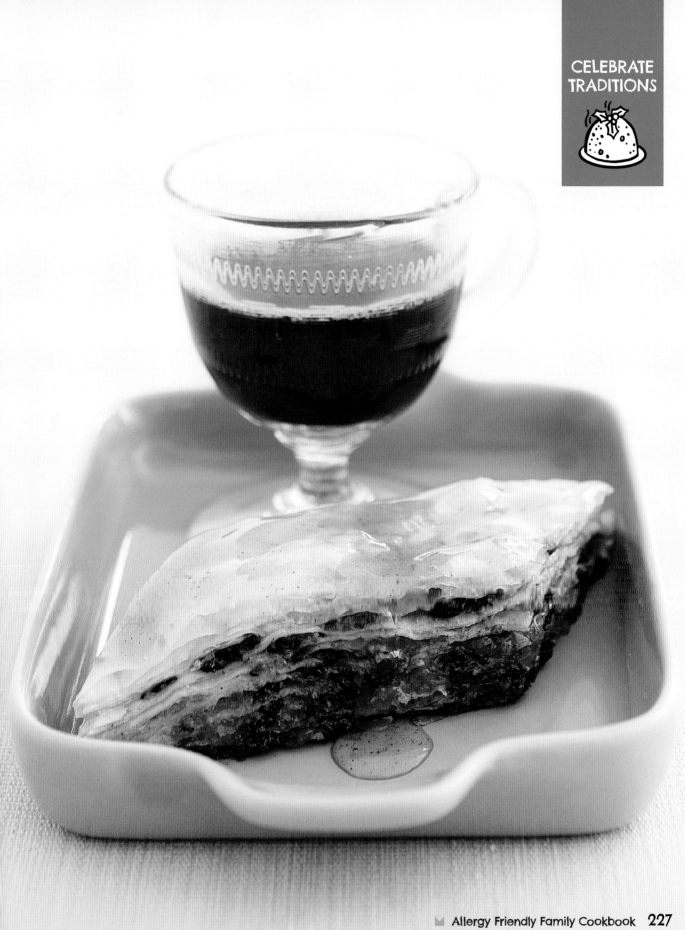

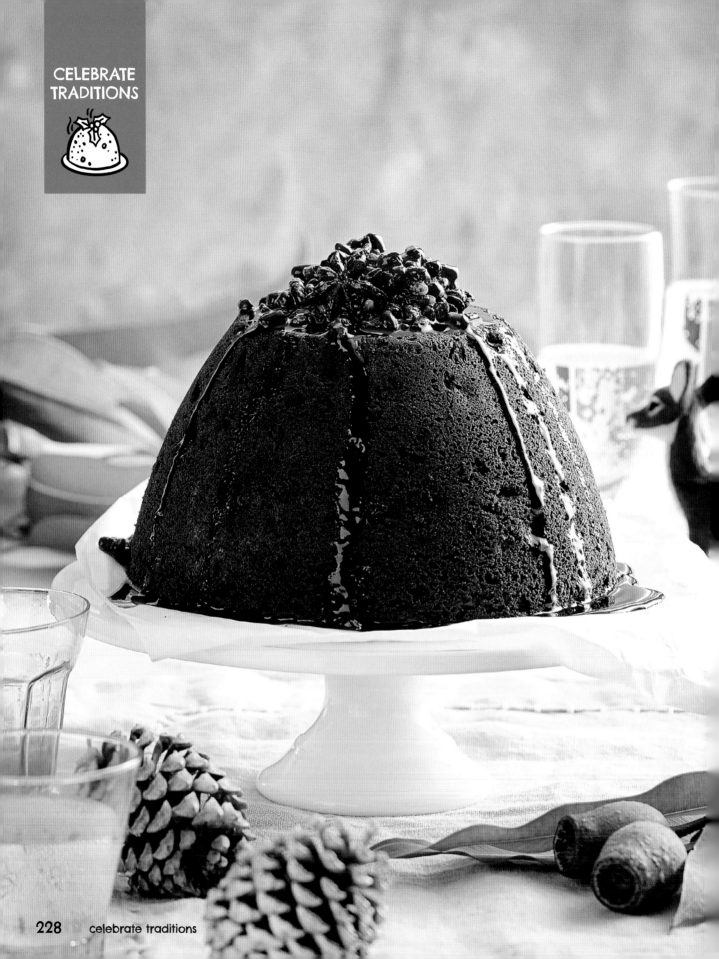

syrupy steamed PUDDING

For the best gluten-free Christmas pudding ever, you'll need to start the fruit mince one week ahead of serving, but it's well worth it!

serves 8 · prep 20 mins (+ standing & 1 hour cooling) · cook 5 hours 10 mins

ingredients

140g (1 cup) buckwheat flour
2½ tsp baking powder
1 tsp bicarbonate of soda
100g (1 cup) almond meal
1 quantity fruit mince
   (see recipe, below)
2 eggs, lightly whisked
125g butter, melted, cooled
80ml (⅓ cup) maple syrup
8 star anise
90g (½ cup) pomegranate arils
Whipped pure cream, to serve

1 Grease a 4L (8 cup) metal pudding steamer with lid. Line base with baking paper. Sift flour, baking powder and bicarb into a large bowl. Stir in almond meal, then fruit mince, egg and butter. Spoon into prepared steamer. Smooth surface. Secure lid. Place in a large stock pot. Pour enough boiling water into pot to reach halfway up side of steamer. Cover. Bring to the boil over medium heat. Reduce heat to low. Simmer for 5 hours, topping up pot with boiling water as needed.

2 Meanwhile, place the maple syrup, star anise and 1 tbs water in a saucepan over low heat. Bring to a simmer. Simmer for 8-10 minutes or until thickened. Add arils. Simmer for 2 minutes. Let cool for 1 hour.

3 Transfer steamer to a board. Stand for 10 minutes. Remove lid. Turn pudding onto a serving plate. Spoon over syrup. Serve with cream.

PER SERVE 10.2g protein, 21.8g fat (9.3g saturated fat), 86.5g carb, 9.3g dietary fibre, 606 Cals (2535kJ)

Fruit mince Combine 1½ cups sultanas, 1 cup chopped dried pitted dates, ½ cup chopped dried apricots, ½ cup currants, 2 tsp finely grated orange rind, ¼ cup orange juice, ¼ cup brandy, 1½ tsp mixed spice, 1 cinnamon stick, 1 star anise and ½ cup maple syrup in a large jar. Secure lid. Store, stirring every 2 days, in a cool dark place for 1 week to develop flavours.

---

make it your way

DAIRY FREE Swap the butter for dairy-free spread, and serve the pudding with dairy-free whipped cream or ice-cream.

basbousa semolina
SLICE

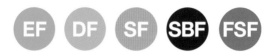

EF **DF** **SF** **SBF** **FSF**

Soaked in a sweet, fragrant syrup, this semolina slice
is popular throughout Eid and Diwali festivities.

serves 24   prep 30 mins (+ cooling & 15 mins resting)   cook 30 mins

ingredients

370g (2 cups) coarse semolina
85g (1 cup) desiccated coconut
215g (1 cup) caster sugar
150g (1 cup) self-raising flour
250ml (1 cup) lemonade
170g (¾ cup) solid coconut oil,
   melted, cooled
24 natural almond kernels

rosewater sugar syrup
315g (1½ cups) caster sugar
1 tsp rosewater essence
1 tsp lemon juice

1 Preheat oven to 200°C/180°C fan forced. Grease a 6cm-deep, 22 x 33cm (base size) roasting pan. Combine the semolina, coconut, sugar and flour in a large bowl. Make a well. Add the lemonade and oil to the well. Stir until combined. Press mixture into prepared pan.

2 Use picture as a guide to cut slice into diamonds. Press 1 almond into the centre of each diamond. Set aside, covered with a tea towel, for 15 minutes to rest. Bake for 30 minutes or until golden.

3 Meanwhile, to make the rosewater sugar syrup, place the sugar and 375ml (1½ cups) water in a small saucepan over low heat. Cook, stirring, for 3-5 minutes or until sugar dissolves. Bring to a simmer. Simmer for 3 minutes or until slightly thickened. Remove from the heat. Stir in rosewater essence and lemon juice.

4 Gradually pour hot syrup evenly over the hot slice, allowing syrup to soak into slice. Cool slice in pan. Re-cut into diamonds. Serve.

PER SERVE 2.4g protein, 9.7g fat (7.8g saturated fat), 37.2g carb, 1.2g dietary fibre, 242 Cals (1014kJ)

make it your way

NUT FREE Simply omit the almonds. You could also use pepitas or raisins, if you like. **GLUTEN FREE** Replace the flour with gluten-free self-raising flour. The cake might become more dense.

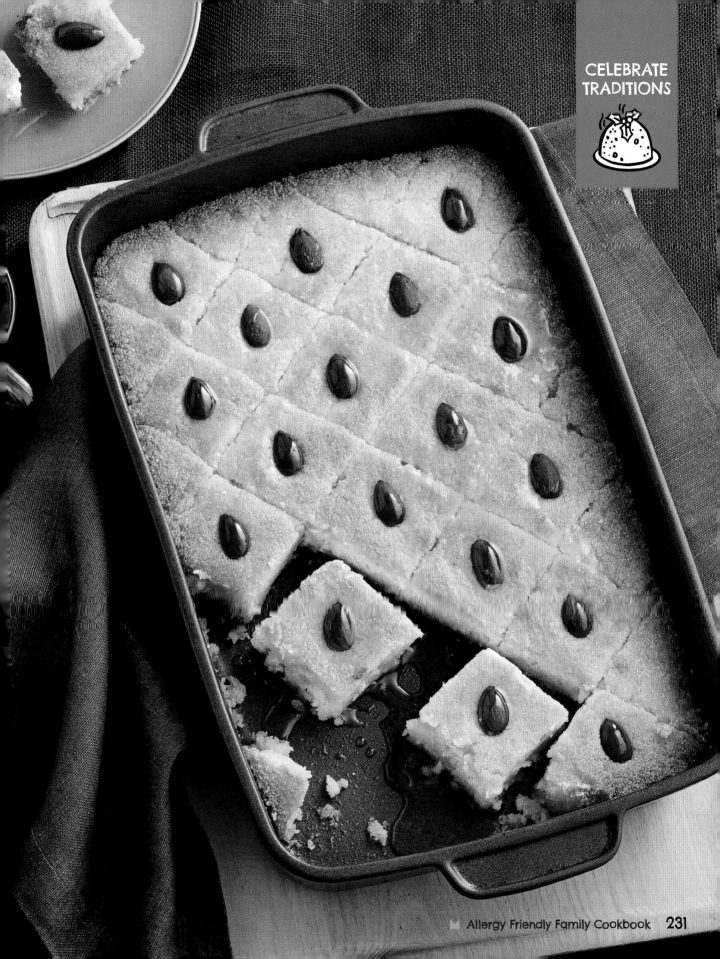

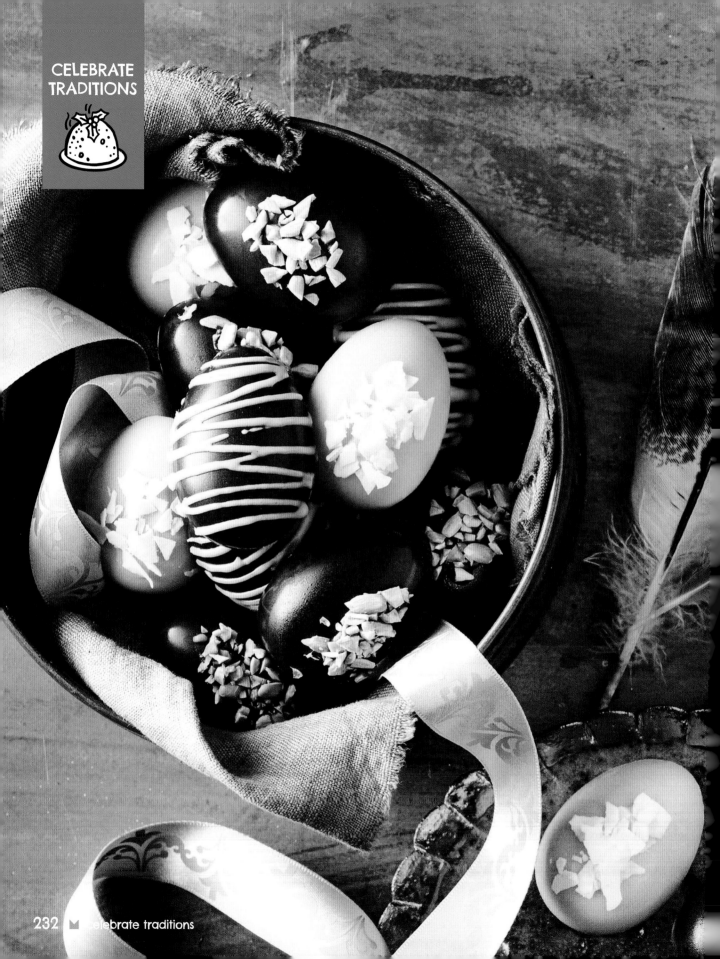

allergy-friendly
EASTER EGGS

The Easter Bunny caters for everyone! These nut- and dairy-free choccy eggs will please kids and adults alike!

makes 8   **prep** 35 mins prep (+ cooling & 15 mins freezing)   **cook** 1 min

ingredients

110g (⅔ cup) sunflower
seed kernels, toasted
1 tbs caster sugar
3½ tsp sunflower oil
½ tsp vanilla extract
¼ tsp ground cinnamon
¼ tsp sea salt
150g dairy-free no-added-sugar
dark chocolate, chopped

1 Reserve 2 tbs sunflower seed kernels. Transfer remaining toasted kernels to a food processor. Add the sugar and process until kernels are finely chopped. Add the oil and process until smooth. Add the vanilla, cinnamon and salt. Process until combined. Transfer to a bowl.

2 Place chocolate in a microwave-safe bowl. Microwave, stirring with a metal spoon halfway through, for 1 minute or until melted and smooth. Stand for 2 minutes to cool slightly. Use a metal spoon to spoon 1 tsp melted chocolate into each hole of an 8-hole (1 tbs) Easter egg mould. Working quickly, use back of the spoon to spread and coat the mould. Freeze for 5 minutes or until firm.

3 Spoon 2 level tsp of sunflower paste into each chocolate shell. Spoon 2 tsp remaining melted chocolate over filling to encase. Freeze for 10 minutes or until firm. Coarsely chop reserved sunflower seeds.

4 Release eggs from moulds. Spread 1 side of eggs with remaining chocolate (reheat to melt, if needed). Sprinkle with chopped seeds. Keep in an airtight container in the fridge until ready to serve.

PER EGG 3.7g protein, 17.9g fat (6.3g saturated fat), 5g carb, 2.8g dietary fibre, 211 Cals (887kJ)

make it your way

SWAP Replace dark chocolate with Caramilk (contains dairy and soy). Use coconut flakes or melted chocolate instead of sunflower kernels.

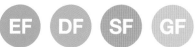

vegan christmas
CAKE

EF **DF** **SF** **GF** **SBF** **FSF**

Start this recipe a week before eating for a fruit cake that will impress and delight. It makes a beautiful gift, too!

serves 20   **prep** 30 mins (+ standing & overnight cooling)   **cook** 2 hours

ingredients

1 quantity fruit mince
   (see recipe, below)
185g Nuttelex spread
2 tbs flaxseed meal
100g (1 cup) almond meal
140g (1 cup) buckwheat flour
45g (⅓ cup) Brazil nuts
45g (⅓ cup) pecan halves
60g (⅓ cup) macadamias,
   halved
40g (¼ cup) pistachio kernels
1½ tbs brandy

1 Preheat oven to 150°C/130°C fan forced. Grease a 7cm-deep, 19cm (base size) square cake pan. Line with 1 layer of brown paper and 2 layers of baking paper, extending paper above edges of pan.

2 Place fruit mince in a large bowl. Discard star anise and cinnamon. Stir in spread. Combine flaxseed and 180ml (¾ cup) water in a jug. Stand for 2 minutes or until thickened. Add to bowl with almond meal and flour. Spread in prepared pan. Decorate top with the nuts.

3 Bake for 2 hours or until a skewer inserted in centre of cake comes out clean. Brush with brandy. Stand for 5 minutes. Turn upside-down onto a tray. Cover with a tea towel. Cool in pan overnight. Serve.

PER SERVE 4.6g protein, 15.5g fat (2.7g saturated fat), 31.9g carb, 4.9g dietary fibre, 301 Cals (1260kJ)

Fig fruit mince Combine 1 cup sultanas, 1 cup dried figs, finely chopped, ½ cup pitted prunes, finely chopped, ½ cup currants, ½ cup dried cranberries, 2 tsp finely grated orange rind, ½ cup brandy, 1½ tsp mixed spice, 1 cinnamon stick, 1 star anise and ⅔ cup firmly packed dark brown sugar in a large airtight container. Secure lid. Store, stirring every 2 days, in a cool dark place for 1 week to develop the flavours.

make it your way

CHANGE PANS Bake for 2 hours in a 7cm-deep, 20cm (base size) round cake pan. Or, bake for 40 mins in an eight-hole (¾ cup) mini loaf pan.

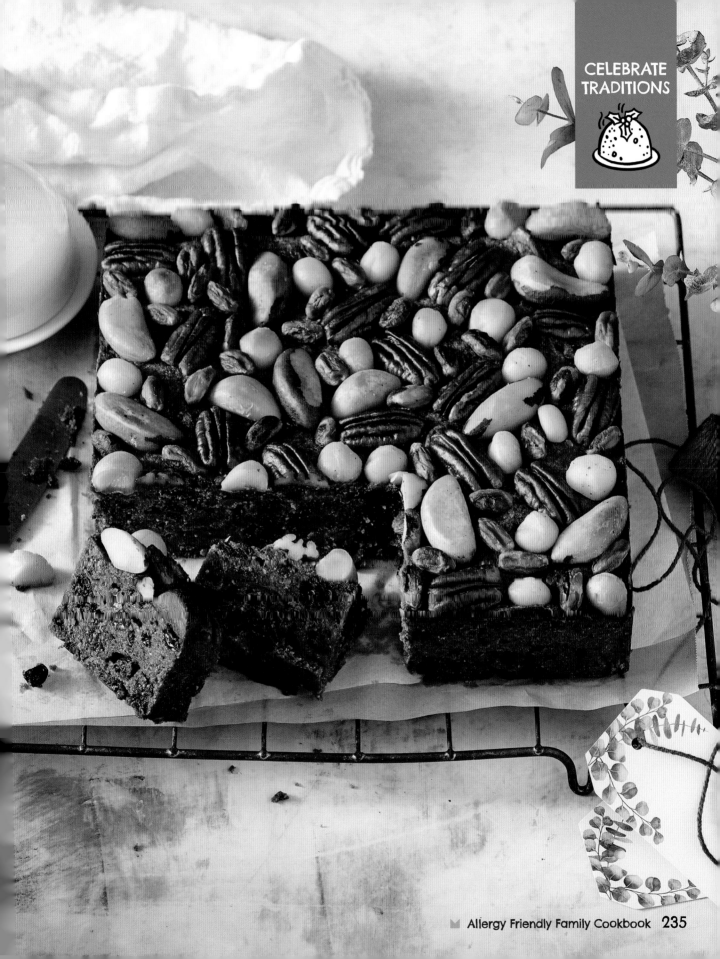

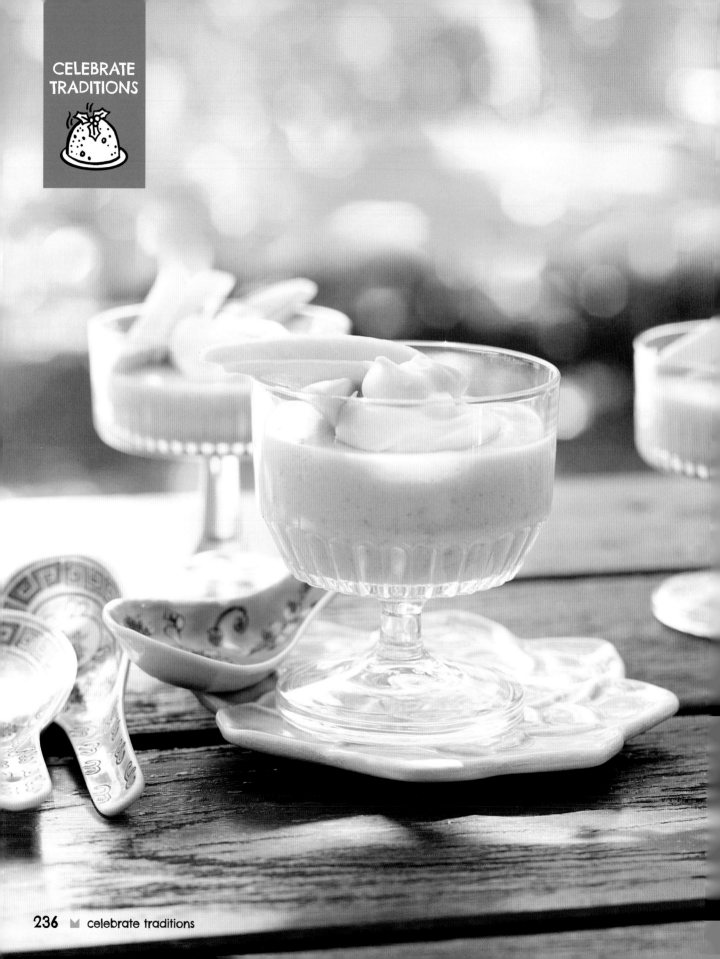

mango
PUDDING

EF · NF · SF · GF · SBF · FSF

Celebrate Chinese New Year with Asian-inspired mango puddings that are quick and easy to make, and quick and easy to eat.

makes 8   prep 20 mins (+ cooling & 6 hours chilling)   cook 5 mins

ingredients

- 2 x 425g cans mangoes in syrup, drained, syrup reserved
- 5 tsp gelatine powder
- 100g (½ cup) caster sugar
- 500ml (2 cups) mango nectar
- 375ml can evaporated milk
- Double cream, and thinly sliced fresh mango (optional), to serve

1 Process canned mango in a food processor until smooth. Transfer to a large bowl. Place 185ml (¾ cup) reserved syrup in a heatproof bowl. Sprinkle with gelatine. Place bowl in a small saucepan. Add enough boiling water to the pan to come halfway up the side of the bowl. Whisk gelatine mixture with a fork until the gelatine dissolves.

2 Place the sugar and 185ml (¾ cup) mango nectar in a saucepan over medium-low heat. Cook, stirring, for 3 minutes or until the sugar dissolves. Set aside to cool.

3 Add gelatine mixture, mango nectar mixture, evaporated milk and remaining mango nectar to the mango puree. Whisk until smooth. Divide among eight 250ml (1 cup) serving glasses. Place in the fridge for 6 hours or until set. Top with the cream and fresh mango, if using, to serve

PER SERVE 7g protein, 15g fat (10g saturated fat), 48g carb, 1g dietary fibre, 351 Cals (1470kJ)

make it your way

DAIRY FREE Use evaporated coconut milk and dairy-free cream.
TRY Top dessert with shaved coconut, or drizzle with mango nectar.

custard dumplings +
HONEY SYRUP

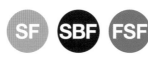

Desserts using semolina, honey and pistachio are a hit during Eid and Diwali. These filo parcels contain all three!

makes 12   prep 35 mins (+ standing & 3 hours chilling)   cook 50 mins

ingredients

55g (¼ cup) caster sugar
330ml (1⅓ cups) milk
½ tsp vanilla bean paste
2 tbs semolina
1½ tbs cornflour
1 egg
8 sheets filo pastry
60g unsalted butter, melted
Coarsely chopped pistachio
  kernels, to serve

spiced honey syrup
215g (1 cup) caster sugar
2 tsp fresh lemon juice
Pinch ground cinnamon
2 tsp honey

1 Combine sugar and 1 cup milk in a saucepan over medium-high heat. Bring to the boil. Remove from heat. Stir in vanilla. Whisk semolina, cornflour, egg and remaining milk in a heatproof bowl until smooth. Slowly add hot milk mixture to semolina mixture, whisking until smooth and combined. Return custard to pan over low heat. Cook, stirring, for 5 minutes or until thickened (do not boil). Spoon into a heatproof bowl. Cover surface with plastic wrap. Place in the fridge for 3 hours.

2 Preheat oven to 180°C/160°C fan forced. Grease a baking tray. Lightly brush 4 filo sheets with melted butter. Stack together. Make 1 more stack. Cut each stack into 6 squares. Heap custard in centre of squares. Bring up sides of filo and pinch firmly to enclose filling. Place on prepared tray. Brush with butter. Bake for 30 minutes or until golden and crisp. Stand for 5 minutes. Place on a heatproof serving platter.

3 To make syrup, combine all ingredients and 125ml (½ cup) water in a saucepan over medium heat. Cook, stirring, for 3 minutes or until sugar dissolves. Simmer, without stirring, for 4-5 minutes or until light golden. Pour over hot dumplings. Sprinkle with pistachios, to serve.

PER SERVE 2.8g protein, 5.7g fat (3.2g saturated fat), 31.9g carb, 0.4g dietary fibre, 167 Cals (700kJ)

make it your way
NUT FREE Leave out the nuts or use chopped sunflower seed kernels.
DAIRY FREE Use dairy-free milk and Nuttelex spread.

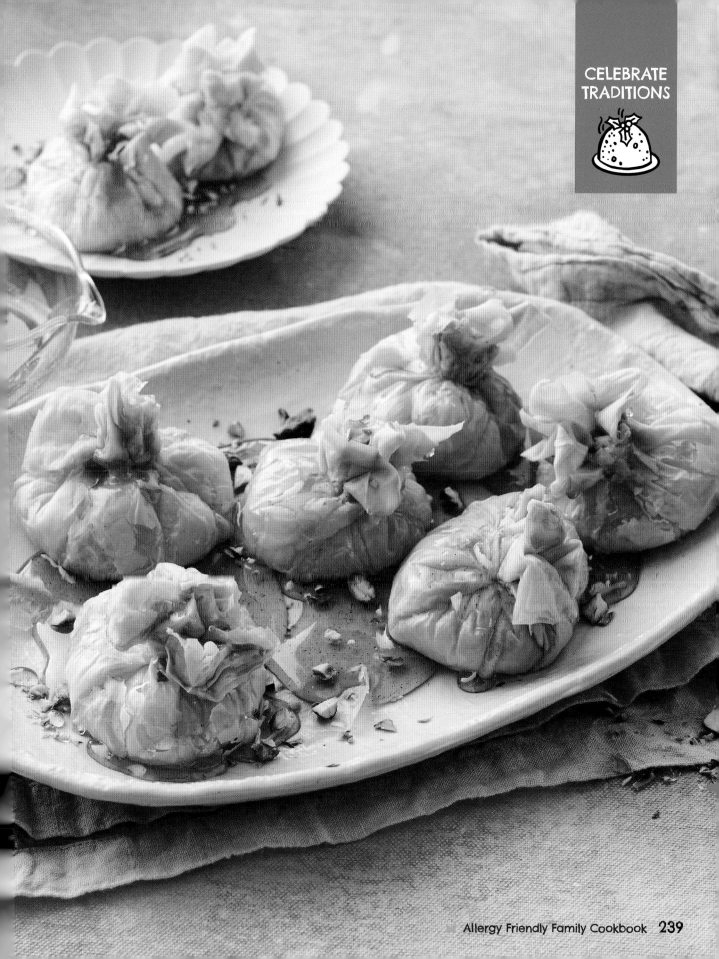

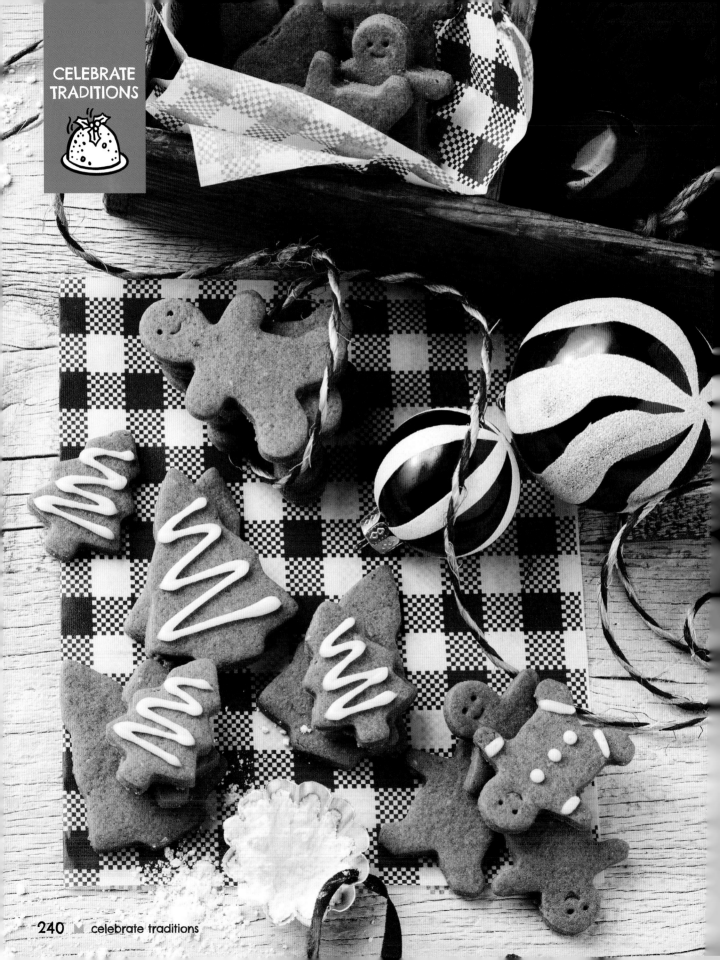

easy vegan
GINGERBREAD

EF DF NF SF SBF FSF

What would Christmas be without gingerbread? Our version uses no eggs or dairy, and are super cute to boot!

makes 26   prep 25 mins (+ 20 mins standing, cooling, 1 hour chilling & overnight setting)   cook 25 mins

ingredients

2 tsp white chia seeds
225g (1½ cups) plain flour, plus extra, to dust
1 tbs ground ginger
1 tsp ground allspice
100g Nuttelex spread
100g (½ cup, firmly packed) dark brown sugar
1 tbs treacle

egg-free royal icing

80g (½ cup) pure icing sugar, sifted
1 tsp glucose syrup
1 tsp fresh lemon juice

1 Combine chia seeds and 1½ tbs water in a bowl. Stand for 20 minutes or until thickened. Sift flour and spices into a bowl. Use fingertips to rub spread into flour mixture until it resembles crumbs. Stir in sugar, treacle and chia mixture. Turn onto a lightly floured surface. Knead until smooth. Shape into 2 discs. Wrap in plastic wrap. Place in fridge for 1 hour.

2 Preheat oven to 180°C/160°C fan forced. Line 2 large baking trays with baking paper. Roll 1 dough disc until 3mm thick. Use a 6.5cm gingerbread man and a 6.5cm Christmas tree cookie cutter to cut out shapes, re-rolling and cutting trimmings as needed. Place 1cm apart on prepared trays. Use a skewer to give gingerbread men eyes and mouths. Bake for 12 minutes or until edges start to brown. Stand on trays for 5 minutes. Transfer to a wire rack to cool. Repeat with remaining dough, using a 5cm gingerbread man and 5cm Christmas tree cookie cutters. Bake for 10 minutes or until edges start to brown.

3 To make royal icing, stir all ingredients and ¾ tsp water in a bowl until smooth. Spoon into a piping bag fitted with a 2mm plain nozzle. Decorate cooled shapes with icing. Leave to set overnight. Serve.

PER PIECE 0.4g protein, 1.1g fat (0.2g saturated fat), 5.5g carb, 0.2g dietary fibre, 33 Cals (137kJ)

make it your way

GLUTEN FREE Swap the flour for gluten-free flour. BOOST Tint some of the royal icing red and green using food colouring.

orange + jelly jack o' LANTERNS

Get into the Halloween spirit and prepare these spooky orange and jelly treats. They're easy and fun to make, and all the kids will just love them.

makes 6   prep 1 hour (+ 3 hours 15 mins chilling)

ingredients
2 x 85g pkts raspberry flavoured jelly crystals
6 large oranges

1 Prepare the jelly mixture following packet directions. Pour into a bowl. Place in the fridge for 15 minutes or until cool but not set.

2 Meanwhile, use a small, sharp knife to cut a 3cm slice from the tops of each orange, and reserve. Cut a very thin slice, making sure not to cut through the pith, from the base of each orange so that it sits flat. Using a spoon, scoop flesh from the oranges (save for another use), leaving only the white pith and the orange rind. Cut a zigzag pattern around the top edge of each orange.

3 Place orange shells on a tray. Pour in enough jelly to fill. Place in the fridge for 3 hours or until the jelly sets.

4 Use a small, sharp knife and picture as a guide to cut the eyes and nose from each orange, making sure you remove the rind and pith, but not the jelly. Replace the orange tops. Serve with a spoon.

PER SERVE 2g protein, 0g fat (0g saturated fat), 25.7g carb, 0g dietary fibre, 107 Cals (448kJ)

make it your way

BOOST Prepare three lots of jelly in red, orange and yellow in 3 separate lamington trays. Once set, cut the jellies into small cubes and combine. Use to fill the oranges.

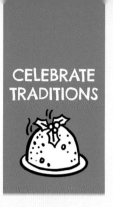
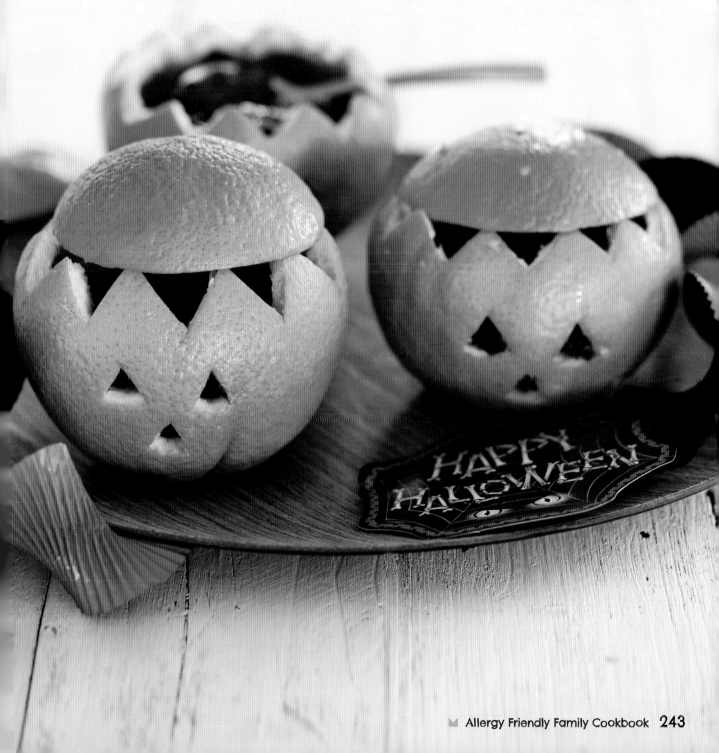

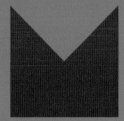

index

Our handy lists are sorted alphabetically, by recipe, allergen and ingredients – making meal selection, shopping and cooking much easier for all!

Allergy Friendly Family Cookbook
ALPHABETICAL INDEX

Looking for a favourite dish or treat? Here's a list of every recipe in this book to make it easier to find the ones you want to try or cook again.

A
Allergy-friendly Easter eggs — 233

B
Banoffee coconut puddings — 177
Basbousa semolina slice — 230
Beef + pumpkin curry — 128
Berry + cherry summer puds — 222
Better-for-you beef stroganoff — 115
Blueberry swirl coconut ice-cream — 161
Bonnie's oat slice — 186

C
Carrot + ginger cupcakes — 215
Cheesy corn + capsicum muffins — 90
Chickpea curry + broccoli rice — 93
Choc-chip cookies — 189
Choc-coconut veganetta — 207
Choc-hazelnut fudge slice — 181
Chocolate + avocado mousse tart — 166
Chocolate birthday cupcakes — 208
Chocolate cherry cake — 199
Chocolate, hazelnut + pear cake — 204
Coconut + strawberry sponge — 203
Coconut eton mess — 182
Coconutty quinoa porridge — 61
Crunchy chocolate granola — 59
Custard dumplings + honey syrup — 238

D
Dairy-free caramel cheesecakes — 165
Dairy-free lasagne — 131
Dairy-free macaroni cheese — 143
Dairy-free Oreo brownies — 173
'Dinosaur egg' meatballs — 151

E
Easy jaffa marble loaf — 154
Easy vegan gingerbread — 241
Egg-free meringues — 178
Eggplant + sweet potato curry — 148

F
Fabulous fish pie — 112
Feta + black bean scrambled eggs — 47
Fig fruit mince — 234
5-minute breakfast bowl — 36
Flourless choc-nut biscuits — 157
Frozen tropical dessert cake — 196
Fruit mince — 229

G
Gluten- + dairy free doughnuts — 170
Gluten-free hot cross buns — 218
Gluten-free prosciutto pizza — 124
Granny's apple crumble — 158
Green goddess sundae — 225
Gulab jamun — 221

H
Ham + corn pasta salad — 73
Healthier tea-time lemon slice — 174
Healthy apricot chicken — 119
Healthy seed crackers — 85
Honey chicken noodle stir-fry — 135

K
Kale + cannellini bean falafels — 74

L
Lauren's cheesecake — 212
Lentil balls in roasted tomato — 144
Loaded gluten-free banana bread — 43
Loaded vegetarian nachos — 132

M
Mac 'n' cheese zucchini slice — 96
Mango pudding — 237
Maple-glazed lamb tray bake — 116
Marvellous mixed berry pancake bake — 60
Masala paste — 148
Mbatata cookies — 185
Mexican polenta muffins — 70
Muffin pan sushi cups — 81

N
Nice 'n' tangy lemon slice — 162
No-bake rawies — 101
Nut-free fruity baklava — 226

O
One-pan baked fried rice — 123
One-pot Mexican beef mince — 140
Orange + jelly Jack o' lanterns — 242
Overnight berry + chia quinoa pots — 39

P
Peri peri chicken lettuce cups — 89
Pie maker cheesy corn fritters — 40
Pie maker zucchini fritters — 78

Q
Quinoa coconut pancakes — 48

R
Raspberry, mint + apple sorbet — 169
Rice paper rolls with chicken — 66

S
Savoury tofu scramble — 56
Simply free apricot bliss balls — 102
Slow-cooked beef dump dinner — 136
Slow cooker honey soy drumsticks — 108
Smoked salmon quiche cups — 82
So good chicken cacciatore — 139
Spiced banana bread — 63
Spicy borlotti bean saltimbocca — 147
Spicy roasted pumpkin soup — 111
Sticky Japanese salmon tray bake — 127
Strawberry-dusted layer cake — 192
Strawberry 'milkshake' cake — 200
Super-quick quinoa bircher — 44
Sweet potato + thyme wraps — 94
Sweet potato, bean + kale shakshuka — 55
Syrupy steamed pudding — 229

T
Teriyaki sushi chicken rice balls — 97
Tuna + avocado sushi salad — 77
Tuna, corn + chive tartlets — 98

U
Ultimate vegan brekky wrap — 52

V
Vanilla birthday cake — 211
Vegan choc-coconut cake — 195
Vegan Christmas cake — 234
Vegan zucchini fritters — 120

W
Wheat-free zucchini slice — 69

Z
Zucchini fritters — 105

Allergy Friendly Family Cookbook
INDEX BY ALLERGEN

Here is our list of recipes featured under each allergy-free icon. Recipes with options (O) allow you to adapt ingredients to cater for an allergy.

EF EGG FREE

Allergy-friendly Easter eggs	233
Banoffee coconut puddings	177
Basbousa semolina slice	230
Beef + pumpkin curry	128
Berry + cherry summer puds	222
Better-for-you beef stroganoff	115
Bonnie's oat slice	186
Carrot + ginger cupcakes	215
Cheesy corn + capsicum muffins (O)	90
Chickpea curry + broccoli rice	93
Choc-chip cookies	189
Choc-coconut veganetta	207
Choc-hazelnut fudge slice	181
Chocolate birthday cupcakes	208
Coconut eton mess	182
Coconutty quinoa porridge	51
Crunchy chocolate granola	59
Dairy-free lasagne	131
Dairy-free macaroni cheese	143
Dairy-free Oreo brownies	173
'Dinosaur egg' meatballs	151
Easy vegan gingerbread	241
Egg-free meringues	178
Eggplant + sweet potato curry	148
Fabulous fish pie	112
Feta + black bean scrambled eggs (O)	47
Fig fruit mince	234
5-minute breakfast bowl	36
Flourless choc-nut biscuits	157
Frozen tropical dessert cake	196
Fruit mince	229
Granny's apple crumble	158
Green goddess sundae	225
Gulab jamun	221
Ham + corn pasta salad (O)	73
Healthier tea-time lemon slice	174
Healthy apricot chicken	119
Healthy seed crackers	85
Honey chicken noodle stir fry	105
Kale + cannellini bean falafels	74

Lauren's cheesecake	212
Lentil balls in roasted tomato	144
Loaded vegetarian nachos	132
Mango pudding	237
Maple-glazed lamb tray bake	116
Marvellous mixed berry pancake bake	60
Masala paste	148
Mbatata cookies	185
Muffin pan sushi cups	81
No-bake rawies	101
Nut-free fruity baklava	226
One-pot Mexican beef mince	140
Orange + jelly Jack o' lanterns	242
Overnight berry + chia quinoa pots	39
Peri peri chicken lettuce cups	89
Quinoa coconut pancakes (O)	48
Raspberry, mint + apple sorbet	169
Rice paper rolls with chicken	66
Savoury tofu scramble	56
Simply free apricot bliss balls	102
Slow-cooked beef dump dinner	136
Slow cooker honey soy drumsticks	108
So good chicken cacciatore	139
Spiced banana bread	63
Spicy borlotti bean saltimbocca	147
Spicy roasted pumpkin soup	111
Sticky Japanese salmon tray bake	127
Strawberry 'milkshake' cake	200
Super-quick quinoa bircher	44
Sweet potato + thyme wraps	94
Sweet potato, bean + kale shakshuka (O)	55
Teriyaki sushi chicken rice balls (O)	97
Tuna + avocado sushi salad (O)	77
Ultimate vegan brekky wrap	52
Vanilla birthday cake	211
Vegan choc-coconut cake	195
Vegan Christmas cake	234
Vegan zucchini fritters	120
Zucchini fritters	105

DF DAIRY FREE

Allergy-friendly Easter eggs	233
Banoffee coconut puddings	177
Basbousa semolina slice	230
Beef + pumpkin curry	128
Berry + cherry summer puds	222
Better-for-you beef stroganoff (O)	115
Blueberry swirl coconut ice-cream	161
Bonnie's oat slice (O)	186
Carrot + ginger cupcakes	215
Cheesy corn + capsicum muffins (O)	90
Chickpea curry + broccoli rice	93
Choc-chip cookies	189
Choc-coconut veganetta	207
Choc-hazelnut fudge slice	181
Chocolate + avocado mousse tart	166
Chocolate birthday cupcakes	208
Chocolate cherry cake	199
Chocolate, hazelnut + pear cake	204
Coconut + strawberry sponge	203
Coconut eton mess	182
Coconutty quinoa porridge (O)	51
Crunchy chocolate granola	59
Custard dumplings + honey syrup (O)	238
Dairy-free caramel cheesecakes	165
Dairy-free lasagne	131
Dairy-free macaroni cheese	143
Dairy-free Oreo brownies	173
'Dinosaur egg' meatballs	151
Easy jaffa marble loaf (O)	154
Easy vegan gingerbread	241
Egg-free meringues (O)	178
Eggplant + sweet potato curry	148
Fabulous fish pie	112
Flourless choc-nut biscuits	157
Fig fruit mince	234
5-minute breakfast bowl (O)	36
Frozen tropical dessert cake	196
Fruit mince	229
Gluten- + dairy-free doughnuts	170
Gluten-free hot cross buns (O)	218

Spooky spider cupcakes n 198
Gulab jamun (O) 221
Ham + corn pasta salad 73
Healthier tea-time lemon slice 174
Healthy apricot chicken 119
Healthy seed crackers 85
Honey chicken noodle stir-fry 135
Kale + cannellini bean falafels 74
Lauren's cheesecake 212
Lentil balls in roasted tomato (O) 144
Loaded gluten-free banana bread 43
Loaded vegetarian nachos (O) 132
Mac 'n' cheese zucchini slice (O) 86
Mango pudding (O) 237
Maple-glazed lamb tray bake 116
Marvellous mixed berry
    pancake bake 60
Masala paste 148
Mbatata cookies 185
Mexican polenta muffins (O) 70
Muffin pan sushi cups 81
Nice 'n' tangy lemon slice (O) 162
No-bake rawies 101
Nut-free fruity baklava (O) 226
One-pan baked fried rice 123
One-pot Mexican beef mince (O) 140
Orange + jelly Jack o' lanterns 242
Overnight berry + chia
    quinoa pots (O) 39
Peri peri chicken lettuce cups 89
Pie maker cheesy corn fritters (O) 40
Pie maker zucchini fritters (O) 78
Quinoa coconut pancakes 48
Raspberry, mint + apple sorbet 169
Rice paper rolls with chicken 66
Savoury tofu scramble 56
Simply free apricot bliss balls 102
Slow-cooked beef dump dinner 136
Slow cooker honey soy drumsticks 108
Smoked salmon quiche cups (O) 82
So good chicken cacciatore 139
Spiced banana bread 63
Spicy borlotti bean saltimbocca (O) 147
Spicy roasted pumpkin soup (O) 111
Sticky Japanese salmon tray bake 127
Strawberry-dusted layer cake 192

Strawberry milkshake cake 200
Super-quick quinoa bircher (O) 44
Sweet potato + thyme wraps 54
Sweet potato, bean + kale shakshuka 55
Syrupy steamed pudding (O) 229
Teriyaki sushi chicken rice balls 97
Tuna + avocado sushi salad 77
Tuna, corn + chive tartlets (O) 98
Ultimate vegan brekky wrap 52
Vanilla birthday cake 211
Vegan choc-coconut cake 195
Vegan Christmas cake 234
Vegan zucchini fritters 120
Wheat-free zucchini slice (O) 69
Zucchini fritters 105

NF NUT FREE

Allergy-friendly Easter eggs 233
Banoffee coconut puddings 177
Basbousa semolina slice (O) 230
Beef + pumpkin curry 128
Berry + cherry summer puds 222
Better-for-you beef stroganoff 115
Blueberry swirl coconut
    ice-cream 161
Burrito bar bites 100
Carrot + ginger cupcakes 216
Cheesy corn + capsicum muffins 90
Chickpea curry + broccoli rice (O) 93
Choc-chip cookies 189
Choc-coconut veganetta 207
Chocolate birthday cupcakes (O) 208
Coconut + strawberry sponge 203
Coconut eton mess (O) 182
Coconutty quinoa porridge (O) 51
Crunchy chocolate granola (O) 59
Custard dumplings
    + honey syrup (O) 238
Dairy-free caramel cheesecakes (O) 165
Dairy-free macaroni cheese (O) 143
Dairy-free Oreo brownies 173
'Dinosaur egg' meatballs 151
Easy vegan gingerbread 241
Egg-free meringues 178
Eggplant + sweet potato curry 148
Fabulous fish pie (O) 112

Fiery + quick lazy
    scrambled eggs (O) 47
Fig fruit mince 204
5-minute breakfast bowl (O) 36
Frozen tropical dessert cake 196
Fruit mince 229
Gluten- + dairy-free doughnuts (O) 170
Gluten-free hot cross buns 218
Green goddess sundae 225
Gulab jamun 221
Ham + corn pasta salad 73
Healthy apricot chicken 119
Healthy seed crackers 85
Honey chicken noodle stir-fry 135
Kale + cannellini bean falafels 74
Lauren's cheesecake 212
Lentil balls in roasted tomato 144
Loaded gluten-free
    banana bread (O) 43
Loaded vegetarian nachos 132
Mac 'n' cheese zucchini slice 86
Mango pudding 237
Maple-glazed lamb tray bake 116
Marvellous mixed berry
    pancake bake 60
Masala paste 148
Mbatata cookies 185
Mexican polenta muffins (O) 70
Muffin pan sushi cups 81
Nut-free fruity baklava 226
One-pan baked fried rice 123
One-pot Mexican beef mince 140
Orange + jelly Jack o' lanterns 242
Overnight berry + chia
    quinoa pots 39
Peri peri chicken lettuce cups 89
Pie maker cheesy corn fritters 40
Pie maker zucchini fritters 78
Quinoa coconut pancakes (O) 48
Raspberry, mint + apple sorbet 169
Rice paper rolls with chicken 66
Savoury tofu scramble 56
Simply free apricot bliss balls 102
Slow-cooked beef dump dinner 136
Slow cooker honey soy drumsticks 108
Smoked salmon quiche cups 82

So good chicken cacciatore 139
Spiced banana bread 63
Spicy borlotti bean saltimbocca 147
Spicy roasted pumpkin soup 111
Sticky Japanese salmon tray bake 127
Strawberry 'milkshake' cake 200
Super-quick quinoa bircher 44
Sweet potato + thyme wraps 94
Sweet potato, bean + kale shakshuka 55
Teriyaki sushi chicken rice balls 97
Tuna + avocado sushi salad 77
Tuna, corn + chive tartlets 98
Ultimate vegan brekky wrap 52
Vanilla birthday cake 211
Vegan choc-coconut cake 195
Vegan zucchini fritters (O) 120
Wheat-free zucchini slice 69
Zucchini fritters 105

SESAME FREE

Allergy-friendly Easter eggs 233
Banoffee coconut puddings 177
Basbousa semolina slice 230
Beef + pumpkin curry 128
Berry + cherry summer puds 222
Better-for-you beef stroganoff 115
Blueberry swirl coconut ice-cream 161
Bonnie's oat slice 186
Carrot + ginger cupcakes 215
Cheesy corn + capsicum muffins 90
Chickpea curry + broccoli rice 93
Choc-chip cookies 189
Choc-coconut veganetta 207
Choc-hazelnut fudge slice 181
Chocolate + avocado mousse tart 166
Chocolate birthday cupcakes 208
Chocolate cherry cake 199
Chocolate, hazelnut + pear cake 204
Coconut + strawberry sponge 203
Coconut eton mess 182
Coconutty quinoa porridge 51
Crunchy chocolate granola 50
Custard dumplings + honey syrup 238
Dairy-free caramel cheesecakes 165
Dairy-free lasagne 131
Dairy-free macaroni cheese 143

Dairy-free Oreo brownies 173
'Dinosaur egg' meatballs 151
Easy jaffa marble loaf 154
Easy vegan gingerbread 241
Egg-free meringues 178
Eggplant + sweet potato curry 148
Fabulous fish pie 112
Feta + black bean scrambled eggs 47
Fig fruit mince 234
5-minute breakfast bowl 36
Flourless choc-nut biscuits (O) 157
Frozen tropical dessert cake 196
Fruit mince 229
Gluten- + dairy-free doughnuts 170
Gluten-free hot cross buns 218
Gluten-free prosciutto pizza 124
Granny's apple crumble 158
Green goddess sundae (O) 225
Gulab jamun 221
Ham + corn pasta salad 73
Healthier tea-time lemon slice 174
Healthy apricot chicken 119
Healthy seed crackers 85
Honey chicken noodle stir-fry 135
Kale + cannellini bean falafels (O) 74
Lauren's cheesecake 212
Lentil balls in roasted tomato 144
Loaded gluten-free banana bread 43
Loaded vegetarian nachos 132
Mac 'n' cheese zucchini slice 86
Mango pudding 237
Maple-glazed lamb tray bake 116
Marvellous mixed berry
  pancake bake 60
Masala paste 148
Mbatata cookies 185
Mexican polenta muffins 70
Muffin pan sushi cups 81
Nice 'n' tangy lemon slice 162
No-bake rawies 101
Nut-free fruity baklava 226
One pan baked fried rice 123
One-pot Mexican beef mince 140
Orange + jelly Jack o' lanterns 242
Overnight berry + chia
  quinoa pots 39

Peri peri chicken lettuce cups 89
Pie maker cheesy corn fritters 40
Pie maker zucchini fritters 78
Quinoa coconut pancakes 48
Raspberry, mint + apple sorbet 169
Rice paper rolls with chicken 66
Savoury tofu scramble 56
Simply free apricot bliss balls 102
Slow-cooked beef dump dinner 136
Slow cooker honey soy drumsticks 108
Smoked salmon quiche cups 82
So good chicken cacciatore 139
Spiced banana bread 63
Spicy borlotti bean saltimbocca 147
Spicy roasted pumpkin soup 111
Sticky Japanese salmon
  tray bake (O) 127
Strawberry-dusted layer cake 192
Strawberry 'milkshake' cake 200
Super-quick quinoa bircher 44
Sweet potato + thyme wraps 94
Sweet potato, bean + kale shakshuka 55
Syrupy steamed pudding 229
Teriyaki sushi chicken rice balls (O) 97
Tuna + avocado sushi salad (O) 77
Tuna, corn + chive tartlets 98
Ultimate vegan brekky wrap 52
Vanilla birthday cake 211
Vegan choc-coconut cake 195
Vegan Christmas cake 234
Vegan zucchini fritters 120
Wheat-free zucchini slice 69
Zucchini fritters 105

GLUTEN & WHEAT FREE

Allergy-friendly Easter eggs 233
Banoffee coconut puddings 177
Basbousa semolina slice (O) 230
Beef + pumpkin curry 128
Berry + cherry summer puds 222
Better-for-you beef stroganoff 115
Blueberry swirl coconut ice-cream 161
Bonnie's oat slice (O) 186
Cheesy corn + capsicum muffins 90
Chickpea curry + broccoli rice 93

Choc-chip cookies 100
Choc-coconut veganetta 207
Choc-hazelnut fudge slice 181
Chocolate + avocado mousse tart 166
Chocolate cherry cake 199
Chocolate, hazelnut + pear cake 204
Coconut + strawberry sponge 203
Coconut eton mess 182
Coconutty quinoa porridge 51
Crunchy chocolate granola 59
Dairy-free caramel cheesecakes 165
Dairy-free lasagne (O) 131
Dairy-free macaroni cheese (O) 143
'Dinosaur egg' meatballs (O) 151
Easy jaffa marble loaf 154
Easy vegan gingerbread (O) 241
Egg-free meringues 178
Eggplant + sweet potato curry 148
Fabulous fish pie 112
Feta + black bean scrambled eggs 47
Fig fruit mince 234
5-minute breakfast bowl 36
Flourless choc-nut biscuits 157
Frozen tropical dessert cake 196
Fruit mince 229
Gluten-free hot cross buns 218
Gluten-free prosciutto pizza 191
Granny's apple crumble 158
Green goddess sundae 225
Ham + corn pasta salad (O) 73
Healthier tea-time lemon slice 174
Healthy apricot chicken 119
Healthy seed crackers 85
Honey chicken noodle stir-fry 135
Kale + cannellini bean falafels 74
Lauren's cheesecake 212
Lentil balls in roasted tomato 144
Loaded gluten-free banana bread 43
Loaded vegetarian nachos 132
Mac 'n' cheese zucchini slice (O) 86
Mango pudding 237
Maple-glazed lamb tray bake 116
Marvellous mixed berry
  pancake bake (O) 60
Masala paste 148
Mbatata cookies (O) 185

Mexican polenta muffins 70
Muffin pan sushi cups 81
Nice 'n' tangy lemon slice 162
No-bake rawies 101
One-pan baked fried rice 123
One-pot Mexican beef mince 140
Orange + jelly Jack o' lanterns 242
Overnight berry + chia
  quinoa pots 39
Peri peri chicken lettuce cups 89
Pie maker cheesy corn fritters 40
Quinoa coconut pancakes 48
Raspberry, mint + apple sorbet 169
Rice paper rolls with chicken 66
Savoury tofu scramble (O) 56
Simply free apricot bliss balls 102
Slow-cooked beef dump dinner 136
Slow cooker honey soy drumsticks 108
Smoked salmon quiche cups 82
So good chicken cacciatore 139
Spiced banana bread 63
Spicy borlotti bean saltimbocca 147
Spicy roasted pumpkin soup 111
Sticky Japanese salmon tray bake 127
Strawberry-dusted layer cake 192
Super-quick quinoa bircher 44
Sweet potato + thyme wraps 91
Sweet potato, bean + kale shakshuka 55
Syrupy steamed pudding 229
Tuna + avocado sushi salad 77
Tuna, corn + chive tartlets 98
Ultimate vegan brekky wrap (O) 52
Vegan zucchini fritters (O) 120
Wheat-free zucchini slice 69
Zucchini fritters (O) 105

🅂🄱🄵 SOY FREE
Banoffee coconut puddings 177
Basbousa semolina slice 230
Beef + pumpkin curry 128
Better-for-you beef stroganoff 115
Blueberry swirl coconut ice-cream 161
Bonnie's oat slice 186
Carrot + ginger cupcakes 215
Cheesy corn + capsicum muffins 90
Chickpea curry + broccoli rice 93

Choc-chip cookies (O) 100
Choc-hazelnut fudge slice 181
Chocolate + avocado mousse tart 166
Chocolate birthday cupcakes 208
Chocolate cherry cake 199
Chocolate, hazelnut + pear cake 204
Coconut + strawberry sponge 203
Coconut eton mess 182
Coconutty quinoa porridge 51
Crunchy chocolate granola 59
Custard dumplings + honey syrup 238
Dairy-free lasagne 131
Dairy-free macaroni cheese (O) 143
'Dinosaur egg' meatballs (O) 151
Easy jaffa marble loaf 154
Easy vegan gingerbread 241
Egg-free meringues 178
Eggplant + sweet potato curry 148
Fabulous fish pie 112
Feta + black bean scrambled eggs 47
Fig fruit mince 234
5-minute breakfast bowl 36
Flourless choc-nut biscuits 157
Frozen tropical dessert cake 196
Fruit mince 229
Gluten- + dairy-free doughnuts 170
Gluten-free hot cross buns 218
Gluten-free prosciutto pizza 191
Granny's apple crumble 158
Green goddess sundae (O) 225
Gulab jamun 221
Ham + corn pasta salad 73
Healthier tea-time lemon slice 174
Healthy apricot chicken 119
Healthy seed crackers 85
Honey chicken noodle stir-fry (O) 135
Kale + cannellini bean falafels 74
Lentil balls in roasted tomato 144
Loaded gluten-free banana bread 43
Loaded vegetarian nachos 132
Mac 'n' cheese zucchini slice (O) 86
Mango pudding 237
Maple-glazed lamb tray bake 116
Marvellous mixed berry
  pancake bake 60
Masala paste 148

Mexican polenta muffins	70
Muffin pan sushi cups	81
Nice 'n' tangy lemon slice	162
No-bake rawies	101
Nut-free fruity baklava	226
One-pan baked fried rice (O)	123
One-pot Mexican beef mince	140
Orange + jelly Jack o' lanterns	242
Overnight berry + chia quinoa pots	39
Peri peri chicken lettuce cups	89
Pie maker cheesy corn fritters	40
Pie maker zucchini fritters	78
Quinoa coconut pancakes	48
Raspberry, mint + apple sorbet	169
Rice paper rolls with chicken (O)	66
Simply free apricot bliss balls	102
Slow-cooked beef dump dinner	136
Slow cooker honey soy drumsticks (O)	108
So good chicken cacciatore	139
Spicy borlotti bean saltimbocca	147
Spicy roasted pumpkin soup	111
Sticky Japanese salmon tray bake (O)	127
Strawberry-dusted layer cake	192
Strawberry 'milkshake' cake	200
Super-quick quinoa bircher (O)	44
Sweet potato + thyme wraps	94
Sweet potato, bean + kale shakshuka	55
Syrupy steamed pudding	229
Ultimate vegan brekky wrap (O)	52
Vanilla birthday cake	211
Vegan choc-coconut cake	195
Vegan Christmas cake	234
Vegan zucchini fritters (O)	120
Wheat-free zucchini slice	69
Zucchini fritters	105

ⓕ FISH & SHELLFISH FREE

Allergy-friendly Easter eggs	233
Banoffee coconut puddings	177
Basbousa semolina slice	230
Beef + pumpkin curry	128
Berry + cherry summer puds	222
Blueberry swirl coconut ice-cream	161
Bonnie's oat slice	186
Carrot + ginger cupcakes	215
Cheesy corn + capsicum muffins	90
Chickpea curry + broccoli rice	93
Choc-chip cookies	189
Choc-coconut veganetta	207
Choc-hazelnut fudge slice	181
Chocolate + avocado mousse tart	166
Chocolate birthday cupcakes	208
Chocolate cherry cake	199
Chocolate, hazelnut + pear cake	204
Coconut + strawberry sponge	203
Coconut eton mess	182
Coconutty quinoa porridge	51
Crunchy chocolate granola	59
Custard dumplings + honey syrup	238
Dairy-free caramel cheesecakes	165
Dairy-free lasagne	131
Dairy-free macaroni cheese	143
Dairy-free Oreo brownies	173
'Dinosaur egg' meatballs	151
Easy jaffa marble loaf	154
Easy vegan gingerbread	241
Eggplant + sweet potato curry	148
Feta + black bean scrambled eggs	47
Fig fruit mince	234
5-minute breakfast bowl	36
Flourless choc-nut biscuits	157
Frozen tropical dessert cake	196
Fruit mince	229
Gluten- + dairy-free doughnuts	170
Gluten-free hot cross buns	218
Gluten-free prosciutto pizza	124
Granny's apple crumble	158
Green goddess sundae	225
Gulab jamun	221
Ham + corn pasta salad	73
Healthier tea-time lemon slice	174
Healthy apricot chicken	119
Healthy seed crackers	85
Kale + cannellini bean falafels	74
Lauren's cheesecake	212
Lentil balls in roasted tomato	144
Loaded gluten-free banana bread	43
Loaded vegetarian nachos	132
Mac 'n' cheese zucchini slice	86
Mango pudding	237
Maple-glazed lamb tray bake	116
Marvellous mixed berry pancake bake	60
Masala paste	148
Mbatata cookies	185
Mexican polenta muffins	70
Muffin pan sushi cups	81
Nice 'n' tangy lemon slice	162
No-bake rawies	101
Nut-free fruity baklava	226
One-pan baked fried rice	123
One-pot Mexican beef mince	140
Orange + jelly Jack o' lanterns	242
Overnight berry + chia quinoa pots	39
Peri peri chicken lettuce cups	89
Pie maker cheesy corn fritters	40
Pie maker zucchini fritters	78
Quinoa coconut pancakes	48
Raspberry, mint + apple sorbet	169
Rice paper rolls with chicken	66
Savoury tofu scramble	56
Simply free apricot bliss balls	102
Slow cooker honey soy drumsticks (O)	108
Smoked salmon quiche cups (O)	82
So good chicken cacciatore	139
Spicy borlotti bean saltimbocca	147
Spicy roasted pumpkin soup	111
Strawberry-dusted layer cake	192
Strawberry 'milkshake' cake	200
Super-quick quinoa bircher	44
Sweet potato + thyme wraps	94
Sweet potato, bean + kale shakshuka	55
Syrupy steamed pudding	229
Teriyaki sushi chicken rice balls	97
Tuna, corn + chive tartlets	98
Ultimate vegan brekky wrap	52
Vanilla birthday cake	211
Vegan choc-coconut cake	195
Vegan Christmas cake	234
Vegan zucchini fritters	120
Wheat-free zucchini slice	69
Zucchini fritters	105

Allergy Friendly Family Cookbook
INDEX BY KEY INGREDIENT

Check out our list of star ingredients - from proteins to vegies, fruit, pasta and chocolate - to make choosing what to cook much easier.

APPLE
Chocolate birthday cupcakes 208
Granny's apple crumble 158
Raspberry, mint + apple sorbet 169

BANANA
Banoffee coconut puddings 177
Choc-chip cookies 189
Loaded gluten-free
　banana bread 43
Spiced banana bread 63

BEEF + LAMB
Beef + pumpkin curry 128
Better-for-you beef stroganoff 115
Dairy-free lasagne 131
Maple-glazed lamb tray bake 116
One-pot Mexican beef mince 140
Slow-cooked beef
　dump dinner 136

BERRIES
Berry + cherry summer puds 222
Blueberry swirl coconut
　ice-cream 161
Chocolate + avocado
　mousse tart 166
Coconut + strawberry sponge 203
Coconut eton mess 182
Egg-free meringues 178
5-minute breakfast bowl 36
Frozen tropical dessert cake 196
Lauren's cheesecake 212
Marvellous mixed berry
　pancake bake 60
Overnight berry + chia
　quinoa pots 39
Raspberry, mint + apple sorbet 169
Strawberry-dusted layer cake 192
Super-quick quinoa bircher 44

CAPSICUM
Cheesy corn + capsicum
　muffins 90
Honey chicken noodle stir-fry 135
Loaded vegetarian nachos 132
Mexican polenta muffins 70
One-pot Mexican beef mince 140
Peri peri chicken lettuce cups 89
So good chicken cacciatore 139
Tuna, corn + chive tartlets 98

CHICKEN
Healthy apricot chicken 119
Peri peri chicken lettuce cups 89
Rice paper rolls with chicken 66
Slow cooker honey soy
　drumsticks 108
So good chicken cacciatore 139
Teriyaki sushi chicken
　rice balls 97

CHOCOLATE
Allergy-friendly Easter eggs 233
Banoffee coconut puddings 177
Choc-chip cookies 189
Choc-coconut veganetta 207
Choc-hazelnut fudge slice 181
Chocolate + avocado
　mousse tart 166
Chocolate birthday cupcakes 208
Chocolate cherry cake 199
Chocolate, hazelnut
　+ pear cake 204
Crunchy chocolate granola 59
Dairy-free Oreo brownies 173
Easy jaffa marble loaf 154
Flourless choc-nut biscuits 157
Green goddess sundae 225
No-bake rawies 101
Vegan choc-coconut cake 195

CITRUS
Easy jaffa marble loaf 154
Healthier tea-time lemon slice 174
Nice 'n' tangy lemon slice 162
Nut-free fruity baklava 226
Orange + jelly Jack o' lanterns 242

COCONUT
Banoffee coconut puddings 177
Basbousa semolina slice 230
Blueberry swirl coconut ice-cream 161
Choc-chip cookies 189
Choc-coconut veganetta 207
Chocolate cherry cake 199
Coconut + strawberry sponge 203
Coconut eton mess 182
Coconutty quinoa porridge 51
Dairy-free caramel cheesecakes 165
Frozen tropical dessert cake 196
Green goddess sundae 225
Healthier tea-time lemon slice 174
Nut-free fruity baklava 226
Quinoa coconut pancakes 48
Simply free apricot bliss balls 102
Spiced banana bread 63
Vegan choc-coconut cake 195

CORN
Cheesy corn + capsicum muffins 90
Ham + corn pasta salad 73
Honey chicken noodle stir-fry 135
Mexican polenta muffins 70
Pie maker cheesy corn fritters 40
Pie maker zucchini fritters 78
Tuna, corn + chive tartlets 98

GRAINS
(OATS, QUINOA)
Coconutty quinoa porridge 51
5-minute breakfast bowl 36

Overnight berry + chia
  quinoa pots   39
Quinoa coconut pancakes   48
Simply free apricot bliss balls   102
Super-quick quinoa bircher   44

LEGUMES
(BEANS, PEAS, LENTILS)
Chickpea curry + broccoli rice   93
Egg-free meringues   178
Feta + black bean
  scrambled eggs   47
Healthy apricot chicken   119
Kale + cannellini bean falafels   74
Lentil balls in roasted tomato   144
Loaded vegetarian nachos   132
Maple-glazed lamb tray bake   116
Spicy borlotti bean saltimbocca   147
Sweet potato, bean +
  kale shakshuka   55
Ultimate vegan brekky wrap   52

MUSHROOM
Better-for-you beef stroganoff   115
Lentil balls in roasted tomato   144
Slow-cooked beef
  dump dinner   136
So good chicken cacciatore   139

PASTA, RICE + NOODLES
Dairy-free macaroni cheese   143
Ham + corn pasta salad   73
Honey chicken noodle stir-fry   135
Lentil balls in roasted tomato   144
Mac 'n' cheese zucchini slice   86
Muffin pan sushi cups   81
One-pan baked fried rice   123
One-pot Mexican beef mince   140
Peri peri chicken lettuce cups   89

Rice paper rolls with chicken   66
Teriyaki sushi chicken rice balls   97
Tuna + avocado sushi salad   77

PORK
(+ HAM, BACON, ETC)
Dairy-free macaroni cheese   143
'Dinosaur egg' meatballs   151
Gluten-free prosciutto pizza   124
Ham + corn pasta salad   73
Mac 'n' cheese zucchini slice   86
One-pan baked fried rice   123
Spicy borlotti bean saltimbocca   147
Wheat-free zucchini slice   69

POTATO
(+ SWEET POTATO)
Eggplant + sweet potato curry   148
Fabulous fish pie   112
Mac 'n' cheese zucchini slice   86
Maple-glazed lamb tray bake   116
Mbatata cookies   185
Slow-cooked beef dump dinner   136
Sticky Japanese salmon
  tray bake   127
Sweet potato + thyme wraps   94
Sweet potato, bean +
  kale shakshuka   55

PUMPKIN
Beef + pumpkin curry   128
Spicy roasted pumpkin soup   111

SEAFOOD
Fabulous fish pie   112
Tuna + avocado sushi salad   77
Tuna, corn + chive tartlets   98
Smoked salmon quiche cups   82
Sticky Japanese salmon
  tray bake   127

SPINACH + KALE
Beef + pumpkin curry   128
Better-for-you beef stroganoff   115
Feta + black bean
  scrambled eggs   47
Kale + cannellini bean falafels   74
Savoury tofu scramble   56
Sweet potato, bean +
  kale shakshuka   55

TOFU
Dairy-free caramel
  cheesecakes   165
Savoury tofu scramble   56

TOMATO
Chickpea curry + broccoli rice   93
Dairy-free lasagne   131
Ham + corn pasta salad   73
Kale + cannellini bean falafels   74
Lentil balls in roasted tomato   144
Loaded vegetarian nachos   132
Savoury tofu scramble   56
Slow-cooked beef dump dinner   136
So good chicken cacciatore   139
Sweet potato, bean +
  kale shakshuka   55
Ultimate vegan brekky wrap   52

ZUCCHINI
Beef + pumpkin curry   128
Better-for-you beef stroganoff   115
Dairy-free lasagne   131
Eggplant + sweet potato curry   148
Mac 'n' cheese zucchini slice   86
Pie maker zucchini fritters   78
Smoked salmon quiche cups   82
Vegan zucchini fritters   120
Wheat-free zucchini slice   69
Zucchini fritters   105

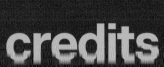

credits

Murdoch Children's Research Institute
project facilitator James Dromey
project coordinator Sarah MacNeill
writer Carolyn Tate
allergy experts Prof Mimi Tang, A/Prof Kirsten Perrett
   and Dr Vicki McWilliams
senior marketing manager Sarah Minogue
senior communications manager Tom Keeble

taste.com.au
editor-in-chief Brodee Myers
executive editor Daniela Bertollo
food director Michelle Southan
creative director Harmony Southern
book art directors Giota Letsios and Chi Lam
book editor Natasha Shaw
book food editor Tracy Rutherford
nutrition editor Chrissy Freer
editorial coordinator Marina Karris

managing director – food and travel Fiona Nilsson

HarperCollinsPublishers Australia
publishing director Brigitta Doyle
publisher Roberta Ivers
editor Shannon Kelly

CONTRIBUTORS
taste.com.au recipes
Alison Adams, Emma Braz, Claire Brookman, Kim Coverdale,
Chrissy Freer, Nadia French, Amira Georgy, Louise Keats,
Liz Macri, Lucy Nunes, Tiffany Page, Louise Patniotis, Kerrie
Ray, Tracy Rutherford, Michelle Southan, Katrina Woodman

Murdoch Children's Research Institute community recipes
Karen Chetner, Kristen Cousins, Lisa Gamble, Catherine
Hornung, Tegan Laird, Sarah MacFarlane, Kat Meldrum,
Frances Oppedisano, Claire Voss

Photography
Guy Bailey, Chris L. Jones, Vanessa Levis, Louise Lister,
Nigel Lough, Sam McAdams-Cooper, Cath Muscat,
Mark O'Meara, Al Richardson, Tracy Rutherford,
Jeremy Simons, Brett Stevens, Craig Wall, Andrew Young

ACKNOWLEDGEMENTS
Murdoch Children's Research Institute exists to give all
children the opportunity to live a healthy and fulfilled life.
From the day the Institute 'opened its doors' in 1986, our
ability to achieve groundbreaking research advances has
been made possible through the time, effort and above all,
trust, of our patients, research participants and their families.
Thank you to all those over the years who have increased
the world's knowledge about allergies – including families
who have taken part in patient surveys, clinical trials or
long-term studies. This book was written not only for,
but ultimately by, you.

We would like to note a special thank you to the Calvort
Jones Foundation whose generous support has assisted in
the publication of this book, which we hope will be of great
benefit to the community. We would also like to specifically
thank News Corp who has been incredibly supportive of
our vision, along with Allergy & Anaphylaxis Australia and
its community who contributed a number of the recipes
you will find in this cookbook, and members of Murdoch
Children's community and staff.

We would also like to acknowledge all the generous
partners and supporters who have, and continue to,
support our allergy research, notably our philanthropic
contributors, research and policy partners, as well as our
many research financial supporters from government.

We hope your family enjoys this book as much as we
enjoyed putting it together for you, and thank you again
for your trust in our work to improve the lives of children
living with allergies. Hopefully this book helps to limit the
stress that childhood allergies can bring to households,
better enabling families to enjoy mealtimes together.

news corp acknowledgements

News Corp Australia and HarperCollins Publishers Australia are proud to support the publication of Murdoch Children's Research Institute's *Allergy Friendly Family Cookbook*.

Since its establishment in 1986, Murdoch Children's has helped solve the illnesses, disorders and myriad other health problems afflicting children all over the world, forging a most distinguished reputation as a world-leading medical research institute.

News Corp has had a long partnership with Murdoch Children's Research Institute, telling the amazing stories of the research, patients and clinicians, sharing some of the great successes of Australia's leading child health research institute, and providing both funding and in-kind support.

We are delighted that our team at Taste has collaborated with Murdoch Children's to produce this valuable book to give children and their families certainty that the food they are eating is free from harm. At News Corp, we believe that working together is key to strong outcomes in child health and it gives us great pleasure to see the work at Murdoch Children's being extended to a much wider audience through this wonderful book.

We have no doubt this book and its recipes are destined to become a kitchen classic.

Through these pages, it is our hope that more people come to learn about Murdoch Children's Research Institute, and its mission-critical work, as leaders in child health.

We are delighted that some of the royalties from this book will go to Murdoch Children's Research Institute to continue its important work.

News Corp Australia is committed to improving the health and wellbeing of all Australians as seen through our long-standing support of child health research.

Thank you to all involved from News Corp Australia, HarperCollins Publishers and Murdoch Children's Research Institute.

We have no doubt this book and its recipes are destined to become a kitchen classic, a mainstay of families across Australia to better cope with the rising problem of food-related allergies. Packed to the brim with full-of-flavour recipes, we know you will find this book useful.

Penny Fowler

Penny Fowler
Chairman Herald and Weekly Times,
News Corp Australia Community Ambassador

HarperCollins*Publishers*
Australia • Brazil • Canada • France • Germany • Holland • India
Italy • Japan • Mexico • New Zealand • Poland • Spain • Sweden
Switzerland • United Kingdom • United States of America

HarperCollins acknowledges the Traditional Custodians of the land upon
which we live and work, and pays respect to Elders past and present.

First published in Australia in 2023
by HarperCollins*Publishers* Australia Pty Limited
Gadigal Country
Level 13, 201 Elizabeth Street, Sydney NSW 2000
ABN 36 009 913 517
harpercollins.com.au

A catalogue record for this book is available
from the National Library of Australia

ISBN 978 1 4607 6285 1 (paperback)
ISBN 978 1 4607 1540 6 (ebook)

Colour reproduction by Splitting Image Colour Studio, Wantirna, Victoria
Printed and bound in China by 1010 Printing

8 7 6 5 4 3 2 1   23 24 25 26